THE ANXIETY CURE: LOVE YOUR BODY

LIVE A LIFE FREE FROM FEAR

CASSANDRA GAISFORD

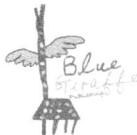

Blue
giraffe

COPYRIGHT

Cover Design by Cassandra Gaisford
Published by Blue Giraffe Publishing 2019

See our complete catalogue on Amazon at Author.to/CassandraGaisford and www.cassandragaisford.com

ISBN PRINT: 978-0-9951137-5-6
ISBN EBOOK: 978-0-9951137-6-3

First Edition

This book is dedicated to love.
And to Lorenzo, my Templar Knight,
who encourages and supports me
to make my dreams possible...
And to all my clients
who have shared their challenges with me,
and allowed me to help make their dreams come true.
Thank you
for inspiring me.

CONTENTS

EXCERPT: MID-LIFE CAREER RESCUE (EMPLOY YOURSELF)

PREFACE

"Nothing beautiful in the end comes without a measure of some pain, some frustration, some suffering."

~ His Holiness the Dalai Lama

"Love what shows up. When you face darkness it dissolves—it only feeds off your denial."

~ Cassandra Gaisford

INTRODUCTION

Are you feeling anxious? Despondent? Stressed or lacking energy? If so, you've come to the right place. It's time to turn up the volume and get your vitality back. But first, it's time to normalize anxiety, depression, and other feelings that impact your mental wellbeing.

As Lady Gaga once said, "There is a lot of shame attached to mental illness, you feel like something is wrong with you…but you can't help it when in the morning you wake up, you are so tired, you are so sad, you are so full of anxiety and the shakes that you can barely think…but (opening up about mental health) was like saying this is a part of me and that's okay."

Low energy is one of the primary ways your

body speaks to you and urges you to make a change.

Life can be incredibly tough—more so, if you're living life raw, not dumbing or numbing your anxiety by escaping into booze, drugs or some other seemingly helpful strategy.

As you'll discover, alcohol and other forms of self-medication only make anxiety worse. Denial and dampening down feelings only deepens wound and worries that crave to be heard, helped, and healed.

Throughout *The Anxiety Cure* you'll find a smorgasbord of helpful, timely strategies. As you'll quickly discover, it's all about proactively embracing healing thoughts and healthy behaviors. Whether it's your mind, body, or soul that needs a lift, you'll see that everything is connected. Even the darkness, despondency, and despair—the joy, the happiness, and radiant bliss.

Without darkness there would be no light. Without winter there would be no summer. Without bad times there would be no happy times. Without some anxiety you'd have nothing to warn you that you need to make a change, restore some balance, or heal a buried part of you.

Sometimes, it can be hard to delve deep, or find ways to bounce back from life-sucking events and toxic people. It can feel as if reclaiming happiness and joy is an impossible dream. Life can knock you around. Sometimes it can feel as though setbacks come in unrelenting waves.

You can feel like you are drowning in a sea of negativity. You can lose hope. If this feels like you, *The Anxiety Cure* comes to your aid. Developing resilience will be some of many helpful tools you'll learn on the way.

We are not born with a fixed, unchangeable amount of resilience. It is a muscle that everyone can build, a skill anyone can master. Armed with new knowledge you can rebound from setbacks. You can learn how to find strength in the face of adversity. And you can build your courage muscles and fire up your determination to live a life of passion, love, and joy.

I'm passionate about helping people find happiness and joy. I know from experience, your health is truly where wealth lies. I genuinely care about your health and well-being. Happier, healthier people contribute to happier, healthier communities.

I hope this book provides some helpful insights and strategies to help you flourish in the wake of any current and future demands you may be experiencing.

You'll find strategies that I've used successfully, personally and professionally to end anxiety, manage stress, and find strength in the face of calamity.

ABOUT THIS BOOK

The Anxiety Cure takes a holistic look at what it takes to create and sustain optimal health. Throughout my counseling and psychology studies, I was so disillusioned and disappointed by the emphasis given to disease and pathologizing those with mental 'illness'.

Frustrated and craving new solutions, I drew my inspiration from the work of leading Māori health advocate and researcher Professor Sir Mason Durie.

Durie created a health and wellness model known as to *Te Whare Tapa Whā*. *Whare*, in Māori, means home, and with its four pillars of health, Durie's model emphasizes the importance of an integrated approach to health and wellbeing.

Twenty or so years ago talk of holistic health,

especially those that integrated spiritual aspects to healing, was considered akin to witchcraft, and certainly not treated seriously. I'm heartened to see conventional practitioners have caught up with what many indigenous people have long known to be true.

Thinking of health as a home is a beautiful way to come back to yourself. To come home—where your heart is. Where you feel safe.

The whare, known as Te Whare Tapa Whā, has four pillars and each wall represents a different dimension of health.

These four pillars are:

- **Taha tinana (physical health)**
- **Taha wairua (spiritual health)**
- **Taha whānau (family health)**
- **Taha hinengaro (mental & emotional health)**

With its strong foundations and four equal sides, it powerfully and simply illustrates the four dimensions of wellbeing that are core to the tools I share throughout *The Anxiety Cure*.

Should one of the four dimensions be missing, neglected, or in some way damaged, a person, or a community, may become 'unbalanced' and subsequently unwell. No doubt you've experienced this yourself—either within your own 'home' or within the larger, extended home of our communities and the world at large.

We know that 40 million people over the age of 18 suffer from anxiety disorders in the United States alone. That statistic alone tells you something is seriously out of balance.

Interestingly, many of my anxious, stressed, or depressed clients who come to counseling or coaching session tell me that one of the things they'd most like to achieve is balance. Yet, in almost all cases they don't know what that means or looks like, or in what areas they are out of balance.

All too often, their nutrition is woeful and exercise seriously lacking (physical health). Similarly, the spiritual dimension is largely neglected or totally ignored. Thoughts and emotions, riddled with stress and anxiety, skew downwards, and relationships are under duress.

Happily, where there's a problem, there's a cure. Worryingly, some statistics suggest only 36.9% of those suffering seek treatment even though anxiety is highly treatable—naturally.

LESS IS MORE

If you've recently picked up this book the chances are you're feeling anxious and perhaps overwhelmed. If you're like me, and many of my clients, less really is more when it comes to digesting information—no matter how beneficial.

For this reason, I've created *The Anxiety Cure* as a four-part series. Each book stands alone and addresses a pillar of health. However, everything is connected. Loving your body can also create beneficial changes in your mind, heart, and soul.

Book One—Love Your Body.
Book Two—Love Your Soul
Book Three—Love Your Feelings
Book Four—Love Your Relationships.

As Buddha once said, "There is a most wonderful way to help living beings overcome grief and sorrow, end pain and anxiety, and realize the highest happiness. That way is the establishment of mindfulness."

Each book in the *The Anxiety Cure* series will help you mind your way to health. Let's take a look at how to bring more mindfulness to our bodies.

LOVE YOUR BODY

So many of us live in our heads and are disconnected from our bodies. We're often aware that both trauma and great healing potential lives within every cell of our body.

Book One, "Love Your Body", reminds and guides you about the importance of caring for your physical health and listening to your body barometer.

If our body is our temple, why do so many of us neglect our physical home? We drive our bodies harder than we drive our cars, and seldom nurture ourselves with preventative and loving self-care.

Fear, panic, irritability, boredom, fatigue, feelings of depression, anger and rage and other joyless experiences are classic signs that it's time for an anxiety cure.

But many people soldier on, ignoring the signs, or self-medicating with booze, drugs, gaming, retail therapy or other distracting addictions. Others feel trapped because they don't know how to make a change for the better.

It takes energy and effort, optimism and feelings of hope and excitement to summon the personal power to transform your life. It also takes a large dose of self-awareness, compassion, and willingness to get to the bottom of your anxiety.

These things can feel in short supply when you're feeling anxious, panicked, discouraged, or so stressed out you can't see the wood for the forest.

The exercises in *Love Your Body* will begin the process of helping you:

• Tune into your body barometer and boost awareness that it's time to change

• Identify the key causes of anxiety and begin identifying a cure

• Fend off panic attacks easily and naturally

• Increase serotonin in your brain without drugs

• Build a strong foundation for change by identifying, and managing toxic stress and building greater resilience

• Gain greater clarity about how and what you want to change and how to direct your energies positively toward your preferred future

• Build hope and confirm there is no better time for you to make a change for the better.

This may be a little book, but the concrete steps and practical tools I share in these pages are powerful solutions regardless of your goals, profession, skills, experience, age, and current situation.

They're a seamless blend of ancient wisdom and modern science. They are timeless and limitless, so it's never "too late" or "too soon" to bounce away from anxiety and despair towards great freedom and joy.

It offers short, sound-bites of stand-alone readings designed to help you cultivate resilience and awareness amid the challenges of daily living.

More than a collection of thoughts for the day, *The Anxiety Cure* offers a progressive program of holistic—mental, emotional, physical and spiritual —study, guiding you through essential concepts, themes, and practices on the path to well-being, joy, and happiness.

The teachings are gently humorous, sometimes challenging, occasionally provocative, but always compassionate and kind, and, I hope, seemingly infinitely wise—and easy to apply.

All that I share are strategies that have worked for me personally through many of my own life challenges, and for my clients in my professional work as a holistic therapist, counselor, and empowerment coach.

The Anxiety Cure features the most essential and stirring passages from my previous books, exploring topics such as: meditation, mindfulness, positive health behaviors, and working with fear, depression, anxiety, and other painful emotions. *The Anxiety Cure* expands upon my previous books in that it encourages a more playful approach to the seriousness of life and the ever-present stressors we all face.

Throughout this book, you will learn practical, creative and simple methods for heightening awareness and overcoming habitual patterns that block happiness and joy and hold you back.

My hope is that next time you are faced with a setback or adversity, one simple phrase will come to mind: "Love what arises." And, having been reminded that bouncing back from setbacks in an accepting and loving manner is the test of your power, that you will then go quickly into resilience mode and apply the strategies you have learned in this book.

If when next faced with a challenge, your default thoughts are 'allow', and 'how can I love what shows up?' then I will consider this book a success.

HOW TO USE THIS BOOK

There is no 'right' or 'wrong' way to work with *The Anxiety Cure*. It's a very flexible tool—the only requirement is that you use it in a way that meets your needs. For example, you may wish to work through the book and exercises sequentially. Alternatively, you may wish to work intuitively and complete the exercises in an ad hoc fashion. Or just start where you need to start.

Each chapter can be read independently. You may wish to read a chapter each week, fortnight or month. Or you may wish to use your intuition and select a page at random, or simply follow your curiosity.

Web links throughout the book and the supplementary resources will help encourage further moments of insight, inspiration, and clarity about the anxiety cure that's right for you.

EXTRA SUPPORT: THE ANXIETY CURE COMPANION WORKBOOK

The Anxiety Cure (the book) offers you information about overcoming anxiety, building resilience and finding joy. Reading a book is great but applying the teachings and writing things down in a dedicated space helps bring the learning alive, deepens your self-awareness, and enables you to make real-world change.

Reading gives you knowledge, but reflecting upon and applying that knowledge creates true empowerment. By writing and recording your responses you're rewriting the story of your life.

As Seth Godin states, "Here's the thing: The book that will most change your life is the book you write. The act of writing things down, of justifying your actions, of being cogent and clear, and forthright—that's how you change."

The Anxiety Cure Companion Workbook will support you through the learning and show you how to create real and meaningful change in your life...simply and joyfully.

So... are you ready? Are you ready to dramatically improve your happiness, success and personal fulfillment? If you've come this far, I think you are...

Let's get going...

AUTHOR'S NOTE

It always really touches me when I realize that what I do has an impact on people. We've all been through tough situations. Not many of us escape childhood unscathed. Few of us survive working life or relationships without scars. I work from that experience. If what I say, write, or do inspires people or gives them strength, courage, or hope, I'm over the moon.

Like many of my books, I write to inspire myself. I take issues I am struggling with, or new learnings that have deeply impacted me, and share them in my books.

The Anxiety Cure is one of these books. I'm tempted to say that it's a concise guide to overcoming anxiety and making the most of your life. It is. And it isn't.

As I wrote this book, so many factors which impact anxiety came to light. Many of them are ignored by general practitioners and doctors—the very people many of us go when we're feeling stressed, anxious, or just plain unwell. Some, are viewed skeptically by psychologists and psychiatrists.

Yet times are changing, the old ways aren't working. Prescription medication and pharmaceutical drugs are being consumed in exploding quantities, and still anxiety rates and other mental illnesses are continuing to soar.

Increasingly science is validating what ancient wisdom has been telling us for years. You only have to consider how main-stream meditation, yoga, acupressure, and other holistic therapies have become, to witness the emergence.

The Anxiety Cure is based on clinically-proven techniques and integrates modern science with other healing modalities.

From my own professional and personal experience, I know we can heal ourselves. A great deal many people don't need pills to feel calm, happy, healthy, and inspired. Some do.

I am not against prescription drugs, but what concerns me, as it may you, is that many anxious, stressed, and depressed people are not offered a choice. Nor do they benefit from someone taking an inventory of their life and analyzing the traumatic events or stressors that may be impacting their anxiety levels.

Like Len, who, aged 42, had suffered work-related burnout, and sought relief from his doctor. He was, quite rightly, alarmed that his doctor told him that the only cure was medication. He left his doctor's office empty handed.

Ten years later, a diagnosis of complex trauma, not only made sense, but also provided a roadmap to lasting healing. I'll be sharing more of his story in a book I plan to write called, Leaving Jehovah—Surviving the Cult of Toxic Control and Shame.

Or, Sarah, who'd been taking anti-depressants for years but had noticed her anxiety rates returning and no longer wanted to be on medication. Counseling and engaging in talk-therapy gave a voice to wounds she had repressed. When darkness was brought to light, and armed with new tools of self-care, including meditation and nutrition, her anxiety rates disappeared.

I'm not bagging medication. Not by any means. My purpose in writing *The Anxiety Cure* is to share alternative routes to healing—lasting ones that enable you to be empowered and chose the best course of action for you.

No two people are the same. We have not had the same childhoods, the same school experiences, or workplace trauma. I speak from my own experience—both what has worked for me, and what has worked for my clients.

With over twenty-five years expertise working in therapeutic professions, most lately as a child therapist and relationship counselor, I know what works.

As you'll read in the chapter, "My Story," I've swum through a tsunami of trauma, hurts, and humiliations and drawn on a range of modalities to help me not just survive, but also thrive.

My hope is in reading this book, you will emerge stronger, happier, healthier, and more thankful too.

A large part of my healing has involved following my joy—something you'll learn to discover for yourself in this book.

I use my passion journal to visualize, gain clarity, and create my preferred future—including my health goals. My clients find this works for them too—along with the other strategies I share in *The Anxiety Cure.*

In this era of anxiety and distraction the need for simple, life-affirming, health-enhancing messages is even more important. If you are looking for inspiration and practical tips, in short, sweet sound bites, this guide is for you.

Similarly, if you are a grazer, or someone more methodical, this guide will also work for you. Pick a page at random, or work through the four pillars of health sequentially.

I encourage you to experiment, be open-minded and try new things. I promise you will achieve outstanding results.

Let experience be your guide, as it has been mine. Give your brain a well-needed break. Let go of 'why', and embrace how you *feel*, or how you want to feel. Honor the messages from your intuition and follow your path with heart.

Laura, who at one stage seemed rudderless career-wise, did just that. Workplace stress was a major source of her anxiety. Finding her passion and following her joy sparked a determination to start her own business. She felt the fear and went for it anyway, emboldened by a desire to live and work like those she looked up to. It was that simple.

As with all of my books, many of the examples I share were inspired by true events in my own life. At the time of writing, I recalled one of the first times I trusted the spiritual realm. I was a teenager when my paternal grandmother was channeled by a psychic and my disbelieving and skeptical self was asked, "Your grandmother says you don't believe she is here. But she is holding out a flower, and she is asking, 'Do you remember the jasmine flowers growing over the house?'

I didn't.

But when I drove home, I called into to Araby Lodge, where my grandmother used to live, and where until her death, she bred and trained her beloved horses. At the time my father lived in her house. I asked him, "What is that vine growing over the house?"

I didn't want to tell him anything about what the psychic had said because I was still skeptical and I didn't want to influence the answer. My father said, "Oh, that old jasmine vine? That's been there forever."

My heart nearly leaped out of my chest. It was at that point that I began to believe in spiritual and psychic phenomena, and in time, many years later, to awaken my own gifts. These gifts weren't awakened without considerable anxiety—something I talk more about in the chapter, "Shadow Work."

It's a timely reminder of just how far following my passion and being free to be me has taken me ——the shy girl who was once afraid of being seen and was terrified of her ability to channel.

As I share in many of my books I hope the following quote is as apt for you as it was for me:

"YOUR STAYING IN THE SHADOWS DOESN'T SERVE THE WORLD."

Here's to learning from our anxiety and transforming our lives with passion, joy, and purpose!

MY STORY

I've experienced some horror work experiences during my life and career—everything from toxic shaming, acute bullying, and being physically threatened. As recently as last year, I experienced the ruthless, underhand, malicious tactics of a narcissistic woman who tried to destroy my career.

Unsurprisingly, all of these experiences increased my anxiety levels. Had I not trained to be a therapist and invested so much time and energy in self-care and resilience strategies I'm not sure I could have coped. Many of these strategies, and those that have helped my clients, I share in the pages that follow.

For most of my childhood, and well into my adulthood I suffered from what I now know was social anxiety. For many, many years it remained undiagnosed and untreated. Were it not for the wise counsel of a psychic who encouraged me to turn my wounds into healing by training to become a counselor, I may still be suffering, silently.

The source of my anxiety can be attributed in part to narcissistic abuse and toxic shaming. Some healers have attributed it to a past-life trauma that I carried forward into this life—telling me that I walk the path of jealously and that relationships are my greatest challenges, but also my most powerful avenues of healing.

You may not believe in past lives or reincarnation and you do not need to in order to benefit from the help contained within this book and others in *The Anxiety Cure* series.

But, in the spirit of authenticity, it feels important to share how I have experienced much healing by journeying into the mystery of mysteries—both the body's and the soul's journey. It is for this reason, amongst others that I have devoted a whole book to spiritual health—Book Three, "Love Your Soul."

I learned later in life, and continue to learn, that healing this family trauma and helping others is my soul purpose in this lifetime.

My purpose can be summed up in one word —love.

To help others love and be loved in return, including self-love and valuing ourselves more than the poisons we may have ingested from people, experiences, circumstances, as we go through this life time.

However, it took me many years to find the gift of my anxiety. My hope is that by writing *The Anxiety Cure*, I may speed up this journey for you.

My anxiety was so bad for most of my teens I tried to drink my way to confidence and numb my anxious feelings with alcohol. In fact, for many years I was so acutely self-conscious I wore green foundation under my makeup to try to hide my blushing face. I was also mercilessly body shamed during my childhood and teenage years. Honestly, for so much of my life all I wanted to do was hide. Often I didn't care if I lived or died.

Anxiety will do that to you—until you befriend it and learn what it wants you to know.

When I was planning my wedding in my late twenties, I wanted a table down the back where no one could see me. Have you ever been to a wedding where the bride wanted to hide?

That's why untreated anxiety is so cruel. It can make us want to stay in the shadows. It can prevent us from standing in the light. Anxiety, left unchallenged can deny us from acknowledging our gifts. It can also leave us splintered, in denial or fear or shame, of those aspects of our personality we need to wield from time to time, but have been taught to devalue and deny.

Saying no to denying who we really are and who we truly want to be and showing up, warts and all, reduces anxiety. Self-acceptance and integration of the polarities within us—the light and the dark, the fear and the courage, the sadness and the anger, the anger and the joy, and the other dualities that, unless befriended wage war within—is the road to inner peace.

We'll dive deeper into the value of integrating shadow work in *The Anxiety Cure*.

For many years I didn't live authentically. I tried, somewhat unsuccessfully, to be someone else. I tried to be who others wanted me to be. Sometimes this was an act of self-preservation driven by fear. Often it was a mistaken belief about my value, and the value of my gifts.

As I've shared in many of my other self-empowerment books, I was once told that I had the soul of an artist. Actively discouraged in childhood, for a long time I'd closed off that side of me. I began my career as a bank-teller, then as an accountant, then as a recruitment consultant, followed by more 'business-minded' careers.

Each time I went further and further away from who I truly was and the things that gave me joy.

As you'll discover in *The Anxiety Cure*, reclaiming joy and living on purpose is a powerful antidote for anxiety. It offers holistic, integrated healing on so many levels—mind, body and soul.

Recently, in my early fifties, I was diagnosed with generalized trauma. All I can say is 'Wow! What a relief!'

No wonder life has felt such a struggle.

Generalized trauma is similar to Post Traumatic Stress Disorder, except that rather than being caused by one traumatic event, it covers a multitude of traumatic events.

Essentially, as Dr. Diane Langberg, Clinical Psychologist and Co-Leader of the Global Trauma Recovery Institute says, if you suffer generalized trauma you've effectively been marinated in trauma from an early age.

Talk about toxicity in the body.

I count myself lucky. Which may surprise you. But as you'll discover in *The Anxiety Cure,* when we befriend our anxiety we can find great fulfillment, purpose and joy.

As the Persian poet and philosopher Rumi once said, "Our wounds are where the light comes in."

Light, love, kindness, hope—these positive energies provide the healing balm we all need.

My trauma, my anxiety and my depression has led me to my Dharma or my purpose in life. My

hope is that all that I share in *The Anxiety Cure* will
help you too.

Much love to you

Cassandra

P.S, I invite you to subscribe to my newsletter to be
the first to know when new books in *The Anxiety
Cure* series are released. I'll also be releasing a four-
book-bundle so you can keep the four pillars of
health I discuss in each book in one easy-to-re-
trieve, place.

1

WHAT IS ANXIETY?

Anxiety can feel like cancer—all invasive and equally as disruptive. But it's not cancer. You can't cut it out, section it, or annihilate with chemical warfare. Anxiety is a feeling. It's got plenty to say and very often a lot to teach you.

You can ignore it, befriend at, or tackle it—but you can't repress it for long. Somewhere, somehow your body keeps the score. The best approach is a multifaceted one, as you will discover, in *The Anxiety Cure*.

Shame, guilt, blame, loss, grief, privilege, insecurity, addiction, identity, love—anxiety feeds off them all. Anxiety is part of being human. It tells us we're still standing. It tells us we're still alive.

But too much anxiety, like too much of anything, is toxic to our mind, body, and soul.

WHAT IS ANXIETY?

Definitions of anxiety vary. Anxiety to me is a crawling, ever-circling predator that feeds on fear and devours the things I love. It's an overwhelming feeling of worry and sense of dread that can spiral out of control sometimes. Which is why I put a lot of time and energy into self-care.

Anxiety is the big brother of stress, toxic stress. It's good to know this because, as you'll discover proactively managing your stress levels and engaging in activities that increase resilience can help you tame this bully easily.

Most of us feel worried at some point in our lives and experience situations that can cause us to feel anxious. While the 'right' amount of anxiety can help us perform better and stimulate action, too much anxiety can tip things out of balance.

Feelings of worry or anxiety are part of a healthy emotional experience. Feeling anxious can warn you and urge you to take care. But when it comes to an intense, prolonged experience, anxiety can be excruciating, unbearable and even debilitating.

In the absence of panic attacks, we may think we are just worrying too much. Our struggles of constant worry may be ignored, minimized or dismissed and, in turn, not properly diagnosed, healed or treated. This is also the case for those with undiagnosed trauma.

You may be surprised to learn how dismissing the impact of traumatic events is negatively impacting your anxiety. You may feel as I once did that things that have happened to you are, "normal" and "just a fact of life." You may be heartened to discover that in no way has your life been normal. Sometimes unearthing the truth provides tremendous clarity and healing. It did for me. It will for you.

Actress Glenn Close recently revealed how her childhood gave her 'a kind of Post Traumatic Stress Disorder (PTSD)'. Only in her sixties did she seek help to heal the emotional trauma of being raised within a right-wing religious cult for thirteen years when she was just seven.

"I visited a childhood trauma specialist not too long ago—even at my age which is kind of astounding. But it establishes these trigger points that affect you for the rest of your life," Close revealed in an interview in 2018.

"I think anybody who has gone through any kind of experience like that doesn't't want to be affected by it. I think it really is interesting how deep it runs," she said.

Similarly, a client of mine who had suffered

childhood sexual abuse as a young boy, waited forty years before seeking therapy. He felt so liberated finally purging those wounds and regaining his life.

We'll look more closely at the intersection of trauma and anxiety, and discover strategies to heal in the chapter, *Trauma Triumph.*

SYMPTOMS

Anxiety can quickly spiral out of control and contribute to a range of mental health challenges. The primary source used to classify mental illnesses is provided by the American Psychiatric Association and their Diagnostic and Statistical Manual of Mental Disorders known as the DSM.

Professionals referring to the DSM look for factors like excessive, hindering worry paired with a variety of physical symptoms, then use assessments to make a diagnosis, and rule out other possibilities.

The DSM-5, for example, outlines specific criteria, or symptoms, to help professionals diagnose Generalized Anxiety Disorder (GAD) and, in turn, create a more effective plan of care. While some professionals may prescribe medication, as you'll discover in this book, this is not the only, nor always, effective way to treat anxiety.

When assessing for GAD, clinical professionals are looking for the following:

1. The presence of excessive anxiety and worry about a variety of topics, events, or activities. Worry occurs more often than not for at least 6 months and is clearly excessive.
2. The worry is experienced as very challenging to control. The worry in both adults and children may easily shift from one topic to another.
3. The anxiety and worry are accompanied with at least three of the following physical or cognitive symptoms (In children, only one symptom is necessary for a diagnosis of GAD):

- Edginess or restlessness
- Tiring easily; more fatigued than usual
- Impaired concentration or feeling as though the mind goes blank
- Irritability (which may or may not be observable to others)
- Increased muscle aches or soreness
- Difficulty sleeping (due to trouble falling asleep or staying asleep,

restlessness at night, or unsatisfying sleep)

Many people suffering from GAD also experience the following symptoms:

- Sweating
- Nausea
- Diarrhoea

However, diagnosis can be an imperfect science, and other medical conditions, lifestyle choices (including excessive alcohol consumption, cannabis and drug use, and undiagnosed traumas) can also lead to similar symptoms.

YOUR ANXIETY CURE

If you are struggling with excessive worry, which makes it hard to carry out day-to-day activities and responsibilities or increasingly leads you to feel depressed, some of the solutions that follow may be just the rescue remedy you need.

But like any medicine, you do have to take action.

For example, part of my self-care plan includes

many of the things we'll discuss in *The Anxiety Cure,* including regular:

- Massage
- Talk-therapy or counseling
- Time alone
- Prayer
- Meditation
- Low consumption of alcohol
- Defragging from social media regularly
- Journaling

In the next chapter, we'll look at some of the ways anxiety is treated, including the growing discontent with pharmaceutical attempts to 'cure' anxiety versus natural ways to increase serotonin and other feel-good hormones in the body-brain.

2

TREATING ANXIETY

As Edmund J. Bourne (Ph.D.) writes in the preface to the Third Edition of *The Anxiety & Phobia Workbook,* there have been several noteworthy changes in the treatment of anxiety disorders. A major shift has been "to give prescription medication more preference, especially when anxiety symptoms are in the *moderate* to *severe range.*"

Borne attributes this in part with the increased awareness of "the role of heredity and neurobiology in the *causation* of anxiety disorders."

My personal and professional view is that while medication intervention can be extremely helpful for some, it is should be used with some degree of caution. Part of that caution involves increasing the awareness of how it may be too readily prescribed without a comprehensive analysis of lifestyle or temporary stressors that may be impacting anxiety levels.

And we'll discuss throughout *The Anxiety Cure, how* in our Western culture, so many people drink excessively, use recreational drugs, over-work, bottle up their feelings, lead sedentary lives, don't switch off, endure toxic and narcissistic relationships, have undiagnosed and untreated trauma— and a vast range of other factors that can lead to excessive worry and anxiety.

Even with the best intentions, a 15-minute doctor's visit will seldom unearth these triggers, and certainly won't heal them. Some therapists have suggested in can take up to three months of repeated visits before clients feel comfortable and safe enough to reveal the real sources of their anxiety.

Intimacy takes time. Which explains, in part, why prescription medication has become the drug of choice.

While any approach that relieves suffering should be utilized science has sometimes been at odds with the notion that people can cure themselves.

I'm also increasingly alarmed by the side effects that many of my clients suffer—including depression and suicidal thoughts. Others just feel tired, lethargic, and demotivated. Some become fat.

In the pages that follow, my intent is to provide ideas, strategies, and suggestions that have been helpful for me personally and for my clients. However, as I'm sure you appreciate they are not intended as a substitute for psychotherapy, counseling, or consulting with your physician.

As a holistic therapist and life coach I know there is a wide range of alternative healing approaches that yield remarkable, extremely quick results. It concerns me, and a lot of other health professionals, that too often people turn to anti-anxiety and antidepressant medication, despite research that cites the lower effectiveness and adverse side-effects.

For many people this still appears to be the solution of choice prescribed by many medical professions.

"Pills are cheap," my doctor told me when I asked her why counseling and therapy wasn't recommended to more people. It may be cheap, but worrying about it is not always effective and the side-effects can also do more harm than healing.

MASKING PAIN DOES NOT OFFER LONG-TERM RELIEF

Rather than offer short-term help very often people come to rely on medical prescriptions for decades. In an extract from his book, _Lost Connections: Uncovering The Real Causes of Depression – and the Unexpected Solutions_, Johann Hari, who took antidepressants for 13 years, says masking the pain does not offer long-term relief and calls for a new approach.

"I was a teenager when I swallowed my first antidepressant. I was standing in the weak English sunshine, outside a pharmacy in a shopping centre in London. The tablet was white and small, and as I swallowed, it felt like a chemical kiss," Hari says.

"That morning I had gone to see my doctor and I had told him – crouched, embarrassed – that pain was leaking out of me uncontrollably, like a bad smell, and I had felt this way for several years. In reply, he told me a story.

"'There is a chemical called serotonin that makes people feel good, he said, and some people are naturally lacking it in their brains. You are clearly one of those people. There are now, thankfully, new drugs that will restore your serotonin level to that of a normal person. Take them, and you will be well.'

"At last, I understood what had been happening to me, and why. However, a few months into my drugging, something odd happened. The pain started to seep through again. Before long, I felt as bad as I had at the start.

"I went back to my doctor, and he told me that I was clearly on too low a dose. And so, 20 milligrams became 30 milligrams; the white pill became blue. I felt better for several months. And then the pain came back through once more. My dose kept being jacked up, until I was on 80mg, where it stayed for many years, with only a few short breaks. And still the pain broke back through."

You can read a summary of Hari's views, including his claims of an over-riding profit motive by pharmaceutical companies, in his interview with The Guardian. <u>'Is everything you think you know about depression wrong?"</u>

A good therapist will often share strategies that can help you rebalance the hormones in your brain, or refer you to other health professionals like nutritionists and dieticians.

As you'll discover in *The Anxiety Cure*, there are numerous ways to increase serotonin in your brain without drugs: including meditation, exercise, sunlight, vitamins and other low-cost approaches.

Many of these approaches will save you money, boost your health, help you reduce weight and improve your relationships. One of these strategies—eliminating or cutting back alcohol consumption—is one I discuss in the chapter Mindful Drinking.

Alcohol has been found to significantly reduce serotonin 45 minutes after drinking. As this article in SpiritScience claims, there is also a clear link between alcohol consumption, anger, violence, suicide and other types of aggressive behavior. Aggression is also heavily linked to low serotonin levels and may be due to alcohol's disrupting effects on serotonin metabolism.

In New Zealand, where talk-therapy or counseling was once generously funded by the Government, several years ago this was diverted to the seemingly more (cost) effective method of prescription medicine. Interestingly, in 2019, moves are afoot to rewrite the imbalance and provide more mental health services, including counselling.

As Bourne also notes, "As a counterpoint to prescription medications, there has also been an increased interest in the use of herbs and natural agents to reduce anxiety. I believe these substances can be quite helpful—some more for anxiety, some more for depression—when such problems are in the *mild* to *moderate* range of severity.

HOLISTIC HEALTH

I first met Alice Morris in 1997 when I went in search of something to help alleviate my soaring stress levels. Other recruitment consultants I worked with at the Global Recruitment agency, where I later developed shingles, swore by her holistic healing approach.

Back in the 90s her approach was innovative— considered almost heretical in the eyes of the mainstream medical profession. Now, much of what she offers, including acupuncture, has been scientifically validated and embraced.

Alice, and her multifaceted approach to managing acute anxiety and toxic stress was my first introduction to mind, body, and soul healing.

And it helped. It helped a lot. Especially her massage, acupuncture, and some of the herbs she prescribed for me.

However, as you'll learn in *The Anxiety Cure*, unless the root cause is addressed, i.e. my toxic work situation, Alice's approach, as with any other, just helped me tread water for a little longer.

When my nervous system finally yelled, "Pay Attention," and I developed shingles, I knew I could no longer lie to myself. I knew I had to leave my job. I share my exactly strategy and more of my story in my Mid-Life Career Rescue series of books.

As you'll read from Alice's story, she also left a less than ideal, yet esteemed career, to follow her true calling. I am grateful to Alice—I credit her work with helping me regain control of the reins of my anxiety and to helping me stay alive— restoring me to strength until such time as I could leave.

"My parents wanted me to be secure in my life in China and their expectations like most Chinese parents were for their children to get a good education and get a high position job so I studied accountancy for 5 years and worked for a big wholesale electrical appliance company as a senior accountant, a job position in which I was the envy of many people at the time.

Even though this was a very successful job and I was considered a success I was not happy in doing it.

In 1990 at the age of 29, I decided to move to New Zealand to follow my dream of understanding true health. This was the perfect opportunity to start doing Chinese medicine again. I worked in Auckland for four years doing herbs and acupressure.

In 1995 I set up the Wellington Health

Massage Clinic followed by the Alice Qigong and Acupressure school. I also returned to China frequently from 1996 studying in Xanxi, Fujian, Anhui, Tai Yuan in Qigong, Fung shui, Chinese Astrology and medicine.

In 2007 I completed an advanced two-month course in Beijing on food healing formulas with Professor Liu who has over 270 branches in China and is one of the leading authorities of the ancient Chinese food healing techniques which is having outstanding results in mainland China.

Through this work I found the New Zealand climate and culture was quite different from China so I had to adjust my treatment according to New Zealand conditions and realised that including Herbs, acupressure, and acupuncture is not enough.

I have found peoples health is not just what the traditional healing methods of acupuncture, acupressure and herbs is but far more including their beliefs, what food they eat, their working state, family state, living environment, general health constitution, lifestyle and their time and date of birth (Chinese Astrology).

A holistic approach is a much deeper way of addressing your health."

Throughout *The Anxiety Cure* you'll discover a

range of natural antidepressants and anxiety-reducing strategies. Importantly, you'll learn empowering strategies that will help you be less dependent on the drug companies and more in control of you and your life.

My hope is that in the process you will experience a feeling of profound joy and peace—a 'feeling of being at home' and reclaiming what you once felt was lost, broken, or missing from your life.

But first, let's try and pinpoint just what's making you anxious.

3

WHAT MAKES YOU ANXIOUS?

Sometimes when you name the beast you can tame the beast.

Here are just a few of many things that can increase feelings of anxiety:

- Mounting debt
- Job loss
- Burnout and stress
- Relationship issues
- Conflict at work
- Public speaking
- Exams and performance appraisals
- Bullying
- Toxic people
- Narcissism
- Trauma

- Fear

Here are a few other common culprits:

- Career dissatisfaction (the job itself, overwork)
- Colleagues or bosses at work
- Health (depression, self-image, weight, illness, etc.)
- Environmental (noise, weather, chaos, etc.)
- Toxic work environments
- Financial uncertainty
- Values conflicts
- Uncertainty
- Change (keeping up with technology)
- Information obesity/overload
- Bombardment/decision fatigue
- Cumulative stress
- The political climate/leadership fears

Lifestyle and health choices can also increase feelings of anxiety including:

- Alcohol consumption and drug use
- Poor diet

- Vitamin deficiencies
- Lack of exercise
- Technology use, including phone overuse
- Social media
- Lack of, or disrupted, sleep
- Lack of work-life balance

Chemical imbalances in your brain and gut may also be the culprit. Including too much or too little of:

- Serotonin
- Dopamine
- Norepinephrine
- Noradrenaline
- and other chemicals, hormones and neurotransmitters

If you're wondering if the symptoms you're having are caused by a chemical imbalance, it's important to know that there's quite a bit of controversy surrounding this theory.

In fact, it's been largely refuted by the medical

community. Researchers argue that the chemical imbalance hypothesis is more of a figure of speech.

It doesn't really capture the true complexity of these disorders. In other words, anxiety and other mental disorders aren't simply caused by chemical imbalances in the brain. As I've already highlighted, there's a lot more complexity to them, and there's also a myriad of natural ways to correct any imbalance.

The chemical imbalance theory also doesn't explain how these chemicals become unbalanced in the first place.

As Harvard Medical School reports, there are likely millions of different chemical reactions occurring in your brain at any given time. These are responsible for your mood and overall feelings. It's impossible to tell if anyone truly has a chemical imbalance in their brain at a given time.

The most common evidence used to support the chemical imbalance theory is the effectiveness of anti-anxiety and anti-depressant medications. These medications work by increasing the amounts of serotonin and other neurotransmitters in the brain.

However, just because your mood can be elevated with drugs that increase brain chemicals doesn't mean that your symptoms were caused by a deficiency in that chemical in the first place. It's just as possible that low serotonin levels are just another symptom of depression, not the cause.

There are no reliable tests to identify imbalances in your brain. Firstly, not all neurotransmitters are produced in the brain. Secondly, neurotransmitter levels in your body and brain are constantly and rapidly changing. This makes tests unreliable.

Thyroid and other disorders can also trigger symptoms of anxiety and other mental disorders.

When it comes to anxiety, there are likely many factors at play. As, you'll discover in the next chapter, even some of the most successful people can suffer from, and recover from, crippling anxiety.

4

ANXIETY FOR ALL

Every human being feels anxious at sometime. According to the National Survey of Mental Health and Wellbeing conducted by the Australian Bureau of Statistics anxiety is the most common mental condition in Australia.

Remember, different people are anxious in different ways. Many people think that being anxious only means being nervous, fearful, or tearful.

This isn't true at all. Many anxious people are quiet, withdrawn or reserved. Other anxious people become angry and enraged.

Some people feel they are going insane.

Anxious people come in all shapes, sizes, and ages. You can become anxious at any age and stage of your life.

Some of the most wildly successful and outwardly confident people suffer from anxiety. Lady Gaga, Robbie Williams, Duff McKagan—and other great performers are just some of the many superstars who suffer from this mental illness.

It might, I suggest, surprise people to hear that the charismatic and mega-talented actress and musician Lady Gaga feels anxious about anything. Recently, as I was, she was given a diagnosis of Post Traumatic Stress Disorder. I suspect the more accurate diagnosis would be Complex Trauma, given the many traumatic situations she has experienced.

Gaga says that taming her anxiety and regulating her nervous system takes daily effort.

"So that I don't panic over circumstances that to many would seem like normal life situations. Examples are leaving the house or being touched by strangers who simply want to share their enthusiasm for my music.

I also struggle with triggers from the memories I carry from my feelings of past years on tour when my needs and requests for balance were being ignored. I was overworked and not taken seriously when I shared my pain and concern that something was wrong.

I ultimately ended up injured on the Born This Way Ball. That moment and the memory of it has changed my life forever. The experience of performing night after night in mental and physical pain ingrained in me a trauma that I relive when I see or hear things that remind me of those days.

I also experience something called dissociation which means that my mind doesn't want to relive the pain so I look off and I stare in a glazed over state. My body is in one place and my mind in another. It's like the panic accelerator in my mind gets stuck and I am paralyzed with fear.

When this happens I can't talk. When this happens repeatedly, it makes me have a common PTSD reaction which is that I feel depressed and unable to function like I used to.

It's harder to do my job. It's harder to do simple things like take a shower. Everything has become harder.

Additionally, when I am unable to regulate my anxiety, it can result in somatization, which is pain in the body caused by an inability to express my emotional pain in words."

She engages with various modalities of psychotherapy to manage symptoms of dissociation and PTSD, that threatened to derail her life before she found her vibe tribe which included mental health support.

When the trauma of her high school bullying and sexual assault was left untreated she said it, "later morphed into physical chronic pain, fibromyalgia, panic attacks, acute trauma responses, and debilitating mental spirals that have included the suicidal ideation and masochistic behavior. Okay. I'm done with my list, but that list changed my life. And it changed my life not in a good way."

"I'm telling you this because for me it was too late," she said. "I needed help earlier. I needed mental health care. I needed someone to see not through me or see the star that I'd become but rather see the darkness inside that I was struggling with."

With her health now manageable, she wants to use her experience to make sure it doesn't happen to anyone else.

"I wish I had mental health resources then because although what I have is treatable and can hopefully and will get better over time, if there was preventative mental healthcare accessible to me earlier, I believe it might not have gotten as bad as it did.

I wish there had been a system in place to protect and guide me. A system in place to empower me to say no to things I felt I had to do.

A system in place to empower me to stay away

from toxic working environments or working with people that were of seriously questionable character."

You'll find a plethora of health resources throughout *The Anxiety Cure* series.

5

HOW DOES ANXIETY IMPACT YOU?

Common signs of anxiety can include, fear, headaches, insomnia, tiredness, depression, anger, and irritability.

The body never lies. However, many people soldier on ignoring the obvious warning signs their body is giving them.

When you feel anxious your body overflows with oxygen and adrenaline. Your heart can race. Your body can mimic a heart-attack.

It's easy to worry about these feelings and think you're going to die. But the reality is your body is just trying to protect you from what it thinks is danger, even though you don't need protecting. This is because of the toxic levels of stress in your body.

PHYSICAL SIGNS OF ANXIETY

- Increased heart rate
- Pounding heart
- Sweaty palms
- Elevated blood pressure
- Tightness of the chest, neck, jaw and back muscles
- Headache
- Diarrhea
- Constipation
- Unable to pass urine or incontinence
- Trembling
- Twitching
- Stuttering and other speech difficulties
- Nausea
- Vomiting
- Sleep disturbances
- Fatigue
- Being easily startled
- Shallow, rapid breathing
- Dryness of mouth or throat
- Cold hands
- Susceptibility to minor illnesses
- Itching
- Chronic pain
- Sore eyes

EMOTIONAL SIGNS OF ANXIETY

- Fear
- Tearful
- Impatience
- Frightened
- Moody
- Highs and lows
- Feeling of loss/grief
- Depression
- Anger
- Irritability
- Short-tempered
- Sadness
- Rage
- Being Hyper-Critical

COGNITIVE SIGNS OF ANXIETY

- Racing thoughts
- Forgetfulness
- Preoccupation
- Errors in judging distance/space
- Diminished or exaggerated fantasy life
- Reduced creativity

- Lack of concentration
- Diminished productivity
- Lack of attention to detail
- Orientation to the past
- Diminished reaction time
- Clumsiness
- Disorganization of thoughts
- Negative self-esteem
- Negative self-statements
- Diminished sense of meaning in life
- Lack of control/need for too much control
- Negative evaluation of experiences

BEHAVIORAL SIGNS OF ANXIETY

- Avoidance
- Carelessness
- Under-eating—leading to excessive weight loss
- Over-eating—leading to weight gain
- Aggressiveness
- Increased smoking/starting smoking
- Withdrawal
- Argumentative
- Increased alcohol or drug use
- Listlessness

- Hostility
- Accident prone
- Nervous laughter
- Compulsive behavior
- Impatience
- Agitation

SOCIAL SIGNS OF ANXIETY

- Relationship difficulties
- Increased conflicts
- Marital issues
- Alienation/withdrawal
- Domestic violence
- Alcohol and substance abuse

SPIRITUAL SIGNS OF ANXIETY

- Hopelessness
- Doubting of values and beliefs
- Withdrawing from fellowship or group support
- Decreased spiritual practices (i.e. prayer, meditation, yoga etc)
- Becoming angry or bitter at a higher power or God

- Loss of compassion —for self and others

It's important to make yourself the boss of your body again. Keep an eye out for any warning signs your body barometer may give you in the future.

When you feel calm what do you notice? How does this differ from times when you are anxious? Sometimes you can 'fake it to make it'—by tricking your body to relax, thinking calming thoughts, stimulating energizing emotions, and engaging in spiritually healing techniques you can restore your mind, body, and spirit to calm.

As always, proactive, not reactive, care is the best strategy. Don't wait too long, and keep up the daily wellbeing practices you'll discover throughout this book.

PILLAR 1: PHYSICAL HEALTH— LOVE YOUR BODY

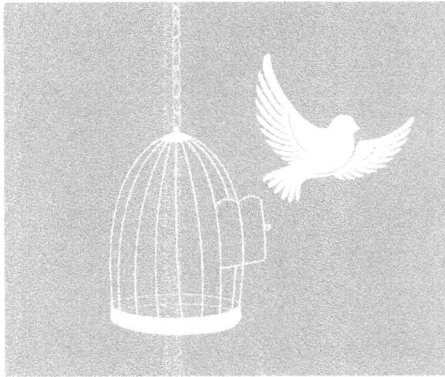

6

YOUR BRILLIANT BODY— NATURAL MOOD-ENHANCING DRUGS

Did you know you have your own drug company? One capable of delivering tremendous relief, and infinitely able to naturally heal anxiety, depression, and a range of other mental imbalances.

Yes, your brilliant body can heal—with a little help.

Serotonin and Dopamine Deficiency

Life is bleak when you are low on serotonin, dopamine and other feel good neurotransmitters. Anxiety, depression, pessimism, and aggression can all come calling.

Thankfully there are natural ways to increase your mood, including:

- Meditation
- Positive thoughts
- Exercise
- Social Dominance
- Sunlight
- Light therapy
- Amino Acids
- Low GI Carbs
- Omega 3
- Gut Bacteria
- Spices—including turmeric
- Limiting or eliminating alcohol

Throughout *The Anxiety Cure: Love Your Body* I'll share a smorgasbord of strategies to reduce anxiety naturally.

I'm not offering a miracle cure, and by no means do I provide an exhaustive list. But I am sharing what's worked for me and the thousands of clients I have helped professionally in my role as a therapist and holistic counsellor.

Best of all many of these strategies are inexpensive and all readily within reach. Many, if not all, are infinitely enjoyable. You'll gain a natural high that keeps on giving.

7

TRAUMA TRIUMPH

Triumphing over trauma is an important part of recovering from anxiety. Few of us get through life without some traumatic experience—often stemming from childhood. Here are just a few of many traumatic life events that have happened to many of my clients, people I have known, and some to me too:

- Parent's divorce
- Sexual assault/rape
- Domestic or family violence
- Community violence (shooting, mugging, burglary, assault, bullying)
- Narcissistic shaming by parents
- Sudden unexpected or violent death of someone close (suicide, accident)

- Abandonment
- Natural disaster such as a hurricane, flood, fire or earthquake
- Poverty and homelessness
- War or political violence (civil war, terrorism, refugee)
- Major surgery or life-threatening illness (childhood cancer)
- Serious injury (burns, dog attack)

Yet so many people don't realize they are one of many walking wounded, and a significant number never seek treatment. I know I didn't, until last year, when I was fifty-three.

Following a particularly toxic and traumatic work experience and a terrifying personal situation I reached out for help and began therapy —again.

Only this time was different. Fate intervened and I was guided to a therapeutic women's circle. The facilitator was a particularly gifted therapist with expertise in healing trauma.

A key part of her approach was helping people acknowledge, verbalize, relive and reintegrate traumatic experiences within their bodies. In this way the trauma was able to be transformed and released.

It was a profoundly healing, empowering, and transformative experience. So much so that I have a renewed focus for my therapeutic work as a counselor and am specializing as a childhood and adulthood trauma specialist.

BODY MEMORIES

Our body is the first thing we disconnect from when we experience trauma. In order to heal, we must first return to the body. The body is the gateway to our awareness.

Very often, as part of our protective mechanism we either blank out or erase memories of traumatic events. As Azita Nahai writes in her terrific book *From Trauma to Dharma*, our bodies are designed to protect themselves from feeling the depths of life's pains until we're ready.

Last year, for example, my mother told me of something that had happened when I was nine-years-old.

"Why can't I remember that?" I asked her. I had absolutely no recollection. Yet, I now realize that this event, along with other traumatic episodes in my childhood remained locked in my body and continued to trigger me.

Leonore Terr (M.D.), Clincial Professor of Psychiatry at the University of California, says that short, single traumas are more likely to be remembered in words. "At any age. however, behavioral memories of trauma remain quite accurate and true to the events that stimulated them."

In other words, while I couldn't verbalize the memory of that trauma, similar events triggered stored experiences, and reactivated my body's stress response.

Even if we do remember the traumatic event, we may try to rationalize, or think our way through issues. We may even try to normalize traumatic situations and may even succeed, yet we still can't make sense of them in our body.

Our minds may lie, but our body always tells the truth.

"Our problem is we numb ourselves from sensing when our bodies truly are ready. They could be screaming at us to finally feel, but we can't hear them," says Nahia.

This was how I was going through my life. With expert guidance my trauma was given a voice in the healing circle. To my surprise, the emotions were waiting for the opportunity to be heard.

Barely into my first hour, it was like the dam burst. Every feeling, every trauma, I hadn't remembered or been ready to feel years prior, every shard of my pain that couldn't be thought or talked about, was there in every fiber of my being. I felt them acutely in my body. And it was all coming up.

I was experiencing all my pain, trauma, and wounds. And beneath the surge and swell of emotions, I felt and heard my body crying out to me.

The ancient Persian poet and philosopher Rumi once wrote that there is a voice that doesn't use words and implores us to listen. And what I heard from the wordless language of my body was this: "Thank you for finally giving me your attention. I've been waiting for you."

And the more I stayed with it, the clearer the message was: When you feel there is something missing in your life, it's probably you. That really was the missing-piece moment for me. On so many levels.

Throughout *The Anxiety Cure,* we'll explore ways to heal the past and exorcize unhelpful emotions that keep you stuck in a cycle of destructive feelings.

As Candace Pert writes in, *Everything You Need to Know to Feel Go(o)d,* "Buried, painful emotions from the past make up what some psychologists and healers call a person's 'core emotional trauma'.

"The point of therapy—including bodywork, some kinds of chiropractic, and energy medicine—

is to gently bring that wound to gradual awareness so it can be re-experienced and understood.

"Only then is choice possible, a faculty of your frontal cortex, allowing you to reintegrate any disowned parts of yourself; let go of old traumatic patterns, and become healed, or whole."

Of course, there are endless ways to get into our bodies, including: yoga, martial arts, tai chi, running, walking, cycling, massage, and other modalities. It's important that you find the path that works best for you.

We are mind, body and soul, and, as you'll discover, it's essential that a physical practice—whatever it may be—also allows a nurturing space to access the spiritual realm, how ever you define it. Spirit, God, Higher Power, Source, Divine, the Universe, Soul, Christ Consciousness, or something else.

8

MINDFUL MEDITATION

His Holiness The Dalai Lama once said, "There is a most wonderful way to help living beings overcome grief and sorrow, end pain and anxiety, and realize the highest happiness. That way is the establishment of mindfulness."

The reason is relatively simple—we're too busy. Our brains never get a break and the results can be increased stress, anxiety, insomnia and if left unchecked, even depression. But there is something you can do—meditate.

Meditation changes brain patterns, soothes and connects you to your Higher Self. It's one of the most powerful bounce strategies you'll ever discover.

"It's the Swiss army knife of medical tools, for conditions both small and large," writes Arianna

Huffington, the founder of *The Huffington Post* and author of *Thrive*.

So, what's the buzz? Recent research published in *New Scientist* has revealed that meditation can help to calm people and reduce fear. The research found that regular meditation can tame the amygdala, an area of the brain which is the hub of fear memory.

People who meditate regularly are less likely to be shocked, flustered, surprised, or as angry as other people, and have a greater stress tolerance threshold as a result.

By meditating regularly, the brain is reoriented from a stressful fight-or-flight response to one of acceptance, a shift that increases contentment, enthusiasm, and feelings of happiness.

Several other beneficial things are going on in your brain. Meditation has been shown in several studies to increase serotonin levels. Serotonin is one of the reasons why we feel peaceful and calm after sitting down and letting go of thoughts.

Meditators also have higher levels of the sleep promoting hormone melatonin. Melatonin is made out of serotonin in the pineal gland—revered by many, including Leonardo da Vinci, as the center of the soul.

You may also enter deep states of bliss and euphoria while you are practicing meditation. This natural high is probably a result of the combination of elevated serotonin and dopamine levels .

Here are a few of the many ways a regular meditative practice will help you:

- Decreased stress and anxiety
- Improved focus, memory, and learning ability
- Heightened recharging capacity
- Higher IQ and more efficient brain functioning
- Increased blood circulation and reduced hyperactivity in the brain, slower wavelengths and decreased beta waves (Beta State:13—30Hz) means more time between thoughts which leads to more skillful decision making
- Increased Theta State (4—8Hz) and Delta States (1—3 Hz) which deepens awareness and strengthens intuition and visualization skills
- Increased creativity and connection with your higher intelligence

When Tim Ferriss, who practices transcendental meditation, sat down with more than 200 people at the height of their field for his new book, *Tools of Titans*, he found that 80% followed some form of guided mindfulness practice.

It took Ferriss a while to get into meditation, he says in a podcast episode about his own morning routine. But since he discovered that the majority of world-class performers meditated, he also decided to follow the habit.

His practice takes up 21 minutes a day: one minute to get settled and 20 minutes to meditate.

Ferriss recommends two apps for those wanting some help getting started—*Headspace* or *Calm*.

"Start small, rig the game so you can win it, get in five sessions before you get too ambitious with length," says Ferriss.

"You have to win those early sessions so you establish it as a habit, so you don't have the cognitive fatigue of that practice."

Many people find that meditating for 20 minutes in the morning and 20 minutes at the end of the day yields remarkable benefits.

Regularly take time to focus on the present moment. Make meditating for at least 20 minutes a day part of your daily routine for optimum success and well-being.

9

JOURNAL YOUR WAY TO JOY

Recently, while tackling a mammoth writing project, I talked myself into a bit of a funk. I knew that what I really needed were some positive reminders of my intentions and a way to encourage perseverance.

I recalled a strategy Anne Gracie, a successful romance author, once shared in a newsletter, "I love my writing journal. It's my partner in writing, there for me whenever I need it, my confidant and my supporter and my record of where I've been."

Prior to this, I had noticed anxiety building—as it always does when I don't have a special book in which to purge and reshape my thoughts.

Instead of saying "I quit" and "I am so over this," and retelling the story that allowed for failure, I went online and purchased a beautiful unlined leather-bound sketchbook.

With my gold pen, I wrote empowering and encouraging quotes from other authors who have also struggled to maintain a prosperous mindset while writing an epic book.

Top of my list was Jessie Burton's empowering words, "Always picture succeeding, never let it fade. Always picture success, no matter how badly things seem to be going in the moment."

These words reminded me that I was picturing failure. I was telling myself messages of failure. I was feeling failure.

Jesse Burton, the author of *The Muse and The Miniaturist*, is very inspiring to me because she is so honest about her own battles with mental health—including anxiety.

"In February, I was publicly honest about how difficult it had been to handle, process and assimilate in real time some of the changes in my life. Namely, the strange and wondrous effects of *The Miniaturist*. I wrote about anxiety, my first tentative foray into putting that mental morass into words," she wrote in one of her newsletters.

As Burton highlights, blogging and sharing your thoughts with your fans is another form of cathartic journaling—as is writing a book like this.

To minimize anxiety and stress and boost your

resilience, another form of journaling is writing Morning Pages, a strategy developed by Julia Cameron, author of *The Artist's Way*.

The writing is just a stream of consciousness, writing out whatever you are feeling—good (or what one of my clients calls the "sunnies") or not so good ("the uglies").

"It's a way of clearing the mind—a farewell to what has been and a hello to what will be," Cameron says.

"Write down just what is crossing your consciousness. Cloud thoughts that move across consciousness. Meeting your shadow and taking it out for a cup of coffee so it doesn't eddy your consciousness during the day."

The point of this writing is to work with your subconscious. and let it work its magic in the creative, healing process.

This strategy, particularly when you use a pen and paper, rather than tap into a keyboard, is profoundly physical. There's something cathartic and freeing about the movement of purging your thoughts on the page, and sweeping them free from your mind.

Another form of journaling is writing a letter to anyone who has wounded you, or who you still feel bitter or angry toward. The point is not to send it, but rather to express feelings that are trapped within your body.

I then recommend burning your painful memories or thoughts in a wonderful ritual or tearing them up. You might find yelling or chanting words of release, adds further depth.

10

HIGH VIBRATION THOUGHTS

Everything is interconnected. Our thoughts affect our bodies as much as what we do with our bodies affects our thoughts.

For example, what you think about affects your serotonin and dopamine levels. A study reported in the Journal of Psychiatry and Neuroscience used positron emission tomography to measure serotonin levels in people who used positive, negative and neutral mood inducing thoughts.

When they reported higher mood levels their serotonin production was higher in the anterior cingulate cortex. When they reported lower mood levels, serotonin production was lower.

This evidence the 2-way traffic of serotonin and mood is 2-way. Serotonin influences mood and mood influences serotonin.

The easiest and quickest way of changing your mood comes from a concept in cognitive neuro-science called Priming.

Priming is using sensory cues to stimulate associations. For example, if you say the word happy, you can't help but get flooded with associations to that word. Automatically you'll probably already think about words, meanings and experiences related to the word happy. Those thoughts alone can cause you to become even happier—literally within seconds.

THINK DOMINATION!

Researchers have also discovered that serotonin production is closely related to hierarchy and social dominance.

Anxiety feeds on fear, low-self worth, and low vibration words. If you want to feel less anxious it's wise to use priming to make yourself more socially confident or dominant.

Words like confident, dominant and strong can trigger feelings associated with serotonin. This is why affirmations are so affective.

You can also change your body language and facial expressions into that of a more socially dominant, less anxious person. Improving your posture, is a simple and effective place to start, as is exercise.

Domination may feel like too strong a word for you—personally, I love the determination and winning attitude that the word evokes.

Whatever words resonate with you, the important thing is to stay positive and not give up on your quest to live anxiety-free. This can also mean learning from your mistakes.

Take a leaf out of Thomas Edison's book. When asked why, after hundreds of unsuccessful attempts at inventing the light bulb, he didn't give up, he replied calmly "I have not failed, I have merely succeeded in finding ways that do not work".

The day before writing this chapter I had a rubbish day. My energy was low and I got distracted and began to feel pessimistic. Instead of staying low I stood back and thought, 'where did I go wrong?' I wrote the following words in my journal that night:

I didn't exercise enough self-care.

I didn't, exercise;

Do my morning pages;

Get outside;

Eat well—other than breakfast I didn't eat anything for the whole day;

Drink *any* water;

Work on my joy project;

Swim in the sea long enough;

Stretch;

Or have the massage I promised myself for completing the hard tasks I'd set.

I also allowed myself to to be dragged along to the launch of a new vodka—and I don't drink. As a result of all the cumulative decisions and actions I had and hadn't made I slept poorly that night. I tossed and turned and began to worry about all the things I had done wrong and hadn't achieved.

It's okay to slip up. It's okay to make mistakes. It's not okay to stop and work out where you got off track—not unless you want to feel anxious. I talk more about the power and life-changing magic of taking responsibility later in this book.

Now is the time to start developing the psychological "muscle" that will get you through any anxiety-inducing behaviors or events.

DEALING WITH UNCERTAINTY

Anxiety feeds on uncertainty. If you haven't set yourself some goals now is the time to do it. Your goals may relate to strategies to show more love to your body and maintain proactive self-care strategies such as regular exercise, meditation and maintaining a better diet.

Setting this renewed commitment will help provide the focus, the momentum, and the reason 'why' to keep you moving forward.

If financial worries are triggering your anxiety you might consider setting goals to trim your expenses, change careers or develop a new source of income on the side.

While checklists and goal setting help, they can't eliminate all uncertainty and risk. The better prepared you are the less anxious you will be. Stay positive and maintain an optimistic outlook.

AFFIRMATIONS: POSITIVE SELF- TALK

Affirmations are statements you can use to give yourself a boost when you experience doubt and uncertainty. When you feel discouraged, try creating your own affirmations or repeating some of the ones below as a way to steady yourself during low times or rough spots.

- "I always achieve my goals"
- "I always achieve whatever I conceive in my mind"

- "I'm gifted and energetic and I believe in myself"
- "I am safe and all is well—everything is working toward my highest good"
- "My perfect role is coming to me now"
- "I deserve the best and people are happy to help me"

Say these affirmations over and over again as many times a day as you need. You will be surprised at how the use of affirmative statements refocuses your energy in a positive way. The following exercise will help you develop your own affirmations.

I keep my affirmations on a digital voice file on my iPhone and play them back after my meditation. I always feel so much more confident and empowered after reinforcing the messages to my higher self reinforced.

Everyone has had negative experiences that cause self-doubt. But our faith in our abilities to accomplish our goals can be reinforced through affirmations. Repeating affirming statements is simply an acknowledgement of what you may already believe but may have come to doubt because of a bad experience.

Think about a situation that might make you

feel uncomfortable, hesitant, or even fearful. Maybe it's making a phone call to a prospective employer to see if they have any vacancies or going for an interview. Or perhaps it's asking someone on a date, or standing up to a bully.

Whatever it might be, imagine yourself experiencing that same difficult situation in a way that you never have before—as your ideal self, confident, self-assured, at ease.

How do look in this fantasy? Describe yourself as you might look and feel:

Pick a few words that describe how you are in your fantasy. Then develop an affirmation using those words to describe yourself in a positive, encouraging way.

Come up with more affirmations to encourage and support yourself.

Repeat the affirmations, eyes closed, putting your trust in the words you have chosen. How do you feel now?

HIGH VIBRATION THOUGHTS

Everything is energy, including your thoughts. Gratitude and appreciation rate highly when it comes to manufacturing feel good vibes.

After completing my journal energy where I berated myself for slipping up on self-care and showing my body some love, I also took time to notice and record what I did well. Anxiety loves to beat us up and tell us we're not good enough.

I did go for a swim. I did tear myself away from my work and spend time with my partner. We danced on a star-lit, sandy beach in American Samoa (where we were holidaying, and where the Vodka launch was being held) as I wrote this chapter.

Remembering these things, even the simple act of going back over past gratitudes, instantly makes me happier. Neuroscientists would tell me that I have successfully manufactured more serotonin and dopamine.

Bravo to me! Bravo to you—because you can do this too.

Other high vibration thoughts are:

- Joy
- Love
- Forgiveness
- Acceptance
- Peace

Low vibration thoughts? I'm sure you know!

- Fear
- Anger
- Hatred
- Doubt
- Anxiety

The list is not exhaustive. To simplify things, given energy is about opposing atoms, think love or fear. Every other emotion is a derivative or variance of them.

Scientific studies, and scientific instruments, can measure the effect of positive and negative thinking and link to the likelihood of disease. Negative thoughts are as powerful as positive ones. Whether you chose positive one or negative ones will result in either high self-esteem or poor self-esteem, happiness or depression, wellness or illness.

How can one person be crippled by a particular event, while another person can thrive in the same situation? It simply comes down to mental attitude!

When you choose a thought—yes, *you do choose* —your brain cells fire up. They vibrate and send off electromagnetic waves. The more you focus on and feed those thoughts, the greater the amplitude of vibration of those cells, and the electric waves, in turn, become stronger.

Positive thinking can raise your vibration up to 10 hertz (Hz), whereas negative thinking can lower your vibration by as much as 15 Hz. These measurements come from Bruce Tainio of Tainio Technology in Cheney, Washington. His company developed new equipment to measure the bio-frequency of humans and foods.

The number one way to start feeling better is to start thinking positively. Choose to love what shows up—no matter what. Love what arises. Fake it until you make it—as I sometimes do when I commit to exercise, or to taking a break, or sometimes even writing. I repeat over and over, "I love this…I'm so happy….this is wonderful—even if I don't believe it. And then I do!

Get to know your default thoughts—the ones that trigger or feed anxiety—and come up with a replacement strategy. I know my default thoughts are, "I'm not good enough." "Whatever I do is not good enough."

Everyday I have to tame them, everyday, even as I write this book, I have to be a warrior and slay them and learn a new language—the language of light and of love.

MOVE!

Exercise reduces anxiety, depression and sensitivity to stress. It is the closest you get to a miracle cure. Validated in numerous psychological studies, moving your body is the single best method of balancing the neurotransmitters in your brain. One of the benefits is that it increases your levels of serotonin naturally.

Exercise also boosts the amount of tryptophan —an essential ingredient in creating serotonin. Best of the all, the mood-elevating effects endure after exercise.

In short, if you want to improve your mood exercise is one of the most important places to start.

Yet so many of us lead sedentary lives. Don't let this be you. Get up and move!

Take heart and encouragement from the many

research studies that have found a reduction in anxiety symptoms with increased physical activity, especially mindful movement, such as yoga, tai chi, and qigong.

For a double-dose of feel good juice consider dance. You know the saying, 'Dance as though no one is watching. Dance as if you've never been hurt.'

Sounds good. Okay, where do I start!

Exercise and movement stimulates the body to produce serotonin and other feel good endorphins, which are chemicals in the brain (neurotransmitters) that help create positive mood. But this only partially explains the positive impacts of exercise.

Exercise can also increase self-esteem, boost self-confidence, enhance social relationships, increase feelings of self-empowerment and control, and other flow-on benefits.

These effects treble when combined with outside energy. Vitamin D sufficiency, along with diet and exercise, has emerged as one of the most important success factors in human health.

BEAT YOUR LOW MOOD

During times of low mood or stress you may become lethargic. Convincing yourself that you don't even have the energy or time to exercise can sabotage your good intentions—increasing feelings of depression and irritability. ..perhaps even guilt.

In the lop-sided state of depression, there is very little electrical activity in your brain. Did you know that a person on a stationary bike has more electrical activity in their brain than a person watching an educational video? Perhaps, even the thought of exercising can have an impact.

But the truly depressed person will have such low electrical activity that making basic decisions, including the mood-enhancing decision to exercise (even just a little), becomes very difficult.

CALM YOUR HYPER-MOOD

Researchers also confirm there is a strong link between breathing, outside energy, and beneficial brainwave patterns. This may explain why so many people say that walking is their meditation—clearing their mind, and allowing space for good ideas to flourish.

Getting up and moving, embracing the flow of 'chi' in your entire system will enable you to activate both hemispheres of your brain—bringing a new perspective as well as greater tolerance to life's stressors.

"It's not that I am thinking but I am in a kind of trance, totally connected with the present moment," Paulo Coelho says. When he returns to his work, his mind is clear and he is more powerfully connected to source energy.

RHYTHM AND FLOW

Some forms of exercise, like swimming, running, cycling or even lifting weights repetitively, helps you get into a rhythmic flow. This repeated action relaxes your mind—and in some cases, creates an almost instantaneous, and often addictive, natural. You've heard people talk about the 'runners high', right? Perhaps you've experienced it for yourself.

Listen to your body barometer when it tells you to exercise more and sloth less. Tune into whether you need fast-stimulating exercise or slow, meditative and gentle.

Either way, commit to a regular exercise regime. Be consistent so that changes easily fall into place and become life-affirming habits.

Discipline yourself to go out and get some fresh air—ideally somewhere not too frenzied.

Combine brisk walking with deep breathing to reduce anxiety, boost your energy levels, short-term memory, and state of mind.

When your breathing is calm and steady, your body is in a nurtured state which helps strengthen your immune system and resilience to stress.

12

LOVE YOUR BED

Are you getting enough sleep? You may need to hit the pillow not the gym.

You can do all the exercise in the world but if you're sleep deprived you'll still be left feeling flat. In fact, lack of sleep is one of the major catalysts to poor mental health.

"We're suffering a sleep crisis," warns Arianna Huffington, co-founder and editor-in-chief of *The Huffington Post* and author of *The Sleep Revolution: Transforming Your Life One Night at a Time*.

Modern science proves conclusively that if you skip out on sleep you're compromising not just your productivity and efficiency, but also your health and wellbeing.

More than a third of American adults are not getting enough sleep on a regular basis, according to a February 2016 study from the Centers for Disease Control and Prevention.

Sleeping less than seven hours a day, they report, can lead to an increased risk of frequent mental distress, impaired thinking, reduced cognitive ability, and increased susceptibility to depression.

Lack of sleep also increases the likelihood of obesity, diabetes, high blood pressure, heart disease, and stroke. None of which will aid your quest for happiness and joy.

Getting enough quality sleep helps you maintain your mental and physical health and enhances your quality of life. Getting enough shuteye helps you keep the world in perspective, and enabling you to refocus on the essence of who you are. In that place of connection, it's easier for the fears and concerns of the world to drop away.

The next time you're worrying and feeling anxious around bedtime, try one of these simple hacks to relax and quieten your mind enough to fall asleep:

- Enjoy a calming cup of herbal tea
- Listen to soothing music
- Read a paperback novel or book of poems

- Take an aromatherapy bath with lavender and other scented oils
- Or, spend time enjoying your favorite relaxation or meditation practice.

You can also enhance your sleep by turning off all devices at least an hour before you go to bed leaving them outside your bedroom.

One of my favorite strategies, and one I often share with my clients, is to train your mind to fall in love with your bed. It may sound strange, but it works. Take Angela for example, a 10-year-old girl who came to see me for help with anxiety-related health issues stemming from bullying at school.

Her anxiety and stress were also accelerated by family dynamics at home, including her older brother recently being expelled from school for smoking cannabis. Her father also suffered from bi-polar disorder and often lost control of his temper.

Angela didn't want to go to bed. She would often wake up and want to see what was going on with the adults in the house. Sometimes, when everyone was getting on, she wanted to sneak a peek at the television.

Her broken sleep spiked her anxiety levels. When she came to see me she had purple and blue rings under her eyes and told me she felt depressed and exhausted.

"I'm afraid of missing out on something," she told me when I asked why she didn't stay in bed. Feeling left out was something she also experienced at school when the bullies ostracized her.

"What do you love about your bed?" I asked. I wanted her to see bed not as a chore, or a punishment, but as something magical—which it is. Quality sleep delivers as many health benefits, if not more, than exercise.

"My bed's so snuggly," she replied.

Amongst other things we talked about, including how lack of sleep was impacting her mood, were the benefits of staying in bed.

I also helped her develop a pampering sleep routine, including aromatherapy. meditation, and having her favorite things around her when she went to bed—including her magical unicorn.

The simple reframe worked. Angela began to look forward to going to bed and staying there. She also developed a routine to help her get in the mood for the bed—something she relished as her sacred time.

As you'll read in the next chapter, "Mood Food," Angela's unicorn was an important part of her therapy.

For other clients, taming their obsession with

social media, and limiting screen time improved their sleep quality and lessened their anxiety considerably.

If lack of sleep is keeping you awake at night and making you tired during the day, consider reading and applying the strategies in Arianna Huffington's book, *The Sleep Revolution: Transforming Your Life One Night at a Time.*

Be ruthless about prioritizing your well-being. Remind yourself of the benefits that will flow when you enhance the length and quality of your sleep.

As you'll read in the next chapter, "Mood Food" when and what you eat can also impact sleep quality and lessen—or spike—anxiety.

13

MOOD FOOD

Diet is an important element of reducing stress and anxiety, particularly when you consider there is at least some biological basis for panic attacks and anxiety.

Increased levels of cortisol , also known as the "stress hormone" are produced during times of stress. This increased level of cortisol can make you crave foods with high levels of salt, sugar and fat.

But eating these foods (or not eating anything at all) can actually elevate your stress levels. Some people crave a quick fix to numb or "medicate" their anxiety, or to get an instant high or energy hit.

Eating too many sugary, 'comfort' foods, drinking too much alcohol or other taking drugs and other substances can trap you in a cycle of short term fixes and longer term anxiety.

Eating lots of processed meat, fried food, refined cereals, candy, pastries, and high-fat dairy products, you're more likely to be anxious and depressed. A diet full of whole fiber-rich grains, fruits, vegetables, and fish can help keep you more balanced

As I shared in my book *Developing a Millionaire Mindset*, successful people make their health a priority and regularly tune into their body barometers.

It's tougher to maintain optimum health behaviors if you lack energy, feel stressed, sluggish, lethargic, or unhealthy. Artificially stimulating your mind, body, and soul won't cut it in the long term.

You are what you feed your stomach—which also feeds your mind. For optimum performance, ensure you're putting smart fuel into your body.

Your gut is also your second brain—a major receptor site of dopamine, a neurotransmitter that helps control the brain's reward and pleasure centers.

Dopamine helps regulate the feel-good emotions we all need to manage anxiety and boost feelings of wellbeing. Dopamine also regulates movement—enabling you to not only see the re-

wards of your efforts, but to also take action towards them.

Benefits of healthy eating practices include:

- Reduced anxiety
- Enhanced mental, emotional, and
  physical health
- Improved mood
- Better sleep
- Increased clarity of thinking
- Better memory
- Healthy body weight
- Increased positive emotions
- More energy and stamina
- Increased determination and goal
  achievement
- Longevity

Avoid extremes—too much sloth makes one
prone to gluttony, too much activity overwhelms,
and too many vain pleasures taken to extremes are
a cause of failure.

Too much coffee, for example, increases feelings of anxiety. Too much sugar, or binge-
drinking booze, as you'll discover in the next
chapters, can send your stress and anxiety levels
soaring.

When you switch from eating unhealthily to

healthily, the difference will be tangibly trans-formative.

Eat small but regular meals to sustain energy levels and keep blood sugar levels steady.

As I mentioned in the previous chapter, "Love Your Bed," Angela's unicorn was an important part of her therapy. She was being bullied at school which lead her to comfort eat and only increased taunting from other children that she was "fat."

In, one session I helped her challenge her thoughts, which is a technique used in Cognitive Behavioral therapy. Taking a blank piece of paper she drew a line. On one side she headed it, *'Nasty Voice,'* and wrote the following words:

Don't eat your lunch—you're too fat.

On the other side of the page, under the heading she had chosen, 'Unicorn—wise voice', she wrote in reply:

Don't listen to that voice. Do what you think is right.

But *Nasty Voice* still had plenty to say:

That voice is wrong. Don't listen.

Unicorn, being the wiser soul, held firm and continued to counsel:

You know what's right, Angela. You've got to eat, or you'll just get sicker.

To end our session we discussed the foods that may add to her anxiety and Angela drew up a list of foods she wanted to avoid and also replaced 'bad foods' with those she liked and was happy to eat. Her list included, *"I love avocado. I love tuna. I love dark green vegetables.*

FOODS AND SUBSTANCES WHICH MAY AGGRAVATE ANXIETY

Caffeine

Of the dietary factors that can aggravate anxiety and trigger panic attacks, caffeine is the most notorious. This includes coffee and caffeinated drinks such as cola and those marketed as 'energy' drinks like V. I go into more detail in the following chapters, *"Avoid Over-Stimulation"* and *"Sweet Misery."*

Stressful Salt

Excessive salt (sodium chloride) stresses the body in several ways: 1) it can deplete your body of potassium, a mineral that's important to the proper functioning of your nervous system and 2) it raises blood pressure, putting extra strain on your heart and arteries.

Consider reducing the amount of salt you consume by avoiding table salt, using a natural salt substitute (such as tamari) both in cooking and on the table, and limiting salty meats, salty snack foods, and other processed foods containing salt as much as possible.

As a guide, it's good to limit your salt intake to one teaspoon per day. If you must buy processed foods, choose those which are labeled low sodium or salt-free.

High-glycemic foods

High-glycemic foods include high-sugar, refined carbohydrates, and processed foods. They cause a rapid rise (and subsequent crash) in blood sugar and destabilize energy levels. Research suggests that high-glycemic foods play a huge role in symptoms of anxiety and depression. High-glycemic types of food make mental health conditions worse, can trigger racing thoughts and panic attacks and should be avoided.

Sugary foods, including biscuits, cakes, candy, and chocolate, and drinks, also promote short-term energy highs, leading to irritability and lethargy.

Preservatives

There are currently about 5000 chemical additives used in the processing of commercial foods. Common artificial preservatives include nitrites, nitrates, potassium bisulfite, monosodium gluta-mate (MSG), BHT, BHA, and artificial colorings and flavorings.

Genetically our bodies are not designed nor equipped to handle these artificial substances. In many cases, very little is known about their long-term biological effects Some have been proven to be carcinogenic (cancer causing) and removed from sale.

Other currently in use, especially monosodium glutamate (found in a lot of Chinese food), nitrites, and nitrates (also found in alcohol), produce al-lergic reactions in many people.

Try to consume unprocessed foods as much as possible and purchase seasonal pesticide-spray-free vegetables grown locally.

Hormones in Meat

Red meat, pork, and most commercially avail-able forms of chicken stem from animals that have been fed hormones to artificially promote weight gain and growth.

Try to replace your consumption of these items with organic raised meats, and fish.

The increasing use of hormones in meat prod-ucts is one of the contributors to increasing num-bers of people turning to a vegan diet. However, take care to ensure you are still receiving optimum levels of key vitamins, including B12.

FOODS WHICH REDUCE ANXIETY

Many studies have been carried out on the link between food and mental health. Making a few diet changes will be helpful. Listed below are some helpful energy-enhancing, mood boosting food tips:

- Eat low-glycemic food such as lean meats, seeds and nuts. Low-glycemic foods are usually low in sugar and high in protein, fiber, and healthy fats. They help stabilize blood sugar levels and help improve mental health. Other examples include vegetables and whole grains
- Meat and fish contain beneficial amounts of iron, as do green leafy vegetables, dried apricots, lentils and other pulses
- Focus on foods high in antioxidants. Most fruits and vegetables are excellent sources of antioxidants, which help fight oxidative stress (cell damage) in your body. Neuropharmacology research suggests that oxidative damage could

play a role in depression and anxiety. High-antioxidant foods include berries, beans, nuts, citrus fruits, and apples.

- Make sure you get sufficient amounts of B-group vitamins, particularly riboflavin, which converts carbohydrates into energy; vitamin B6 essential for energy metabolism; and vitamin B12, is required for forming red blood cells that carry oxygen throughout the body. Vitamin B-complex help to increase your resilience to stress, which can aggravate blood sugar swings. Useful sources of B-group vitamins include wholegrains, chicken, fish, eggs, dairy produce, pulses, shellfish and red meat
- Help your body absorb more iron by drinking a glass of orange juice once a day with a meal. Vitamin C also helps to boost energy and stress resilience.
- Other vital minerals include foods high in magnesium. Magnesium has a calming effect, and deficiency in this mineral could increase and lead to anxiety. Magnesium also works with potassium and sodium to ensure the efficient working of muscles, along with zinc, which protects against viral infections

that often precede chronic fatigue. Good sources of magnesium include spinach, almonds, quinoa, tofu, and black beans.

Don't forget to set your self up for an anxiety-free day by eating a nourishing breakfast. Too many people skip this important start to the day.

At first glance, porridge might not seem like the most exciting breakfast on the planet. But it's great for your health and way better than a greasy fry-up. One bowl of porridge contains more fiber than a slice of wholemeal bread and is rich in minerals including copper, iron, and manganese.

It's also been proven to prevent blood sugar spikes, due to the low glycemic index of oats.

It's easy to miss meals when you're busy or stressed, so plan ahead. Your body, mind and spirit will love you back.

STRESSFUL EATING HABITS

Stress and anxiety can be aggravated not only by what you eat but by the way you eat. In our modern, adrenaline-fueled, fast-paced society, many of us simply do not give ourselves enough time for eating.

Any of the following habits can aggravate your daily level of stress:

- Eating too fast or on the run
- Not chewing food at least 15-20 times per mouthful (your stomach does not have teeth—food must be partially predigested in your mouth for nutrients and enzymes to do their work)
- Over-eating , to the point of feeling stuffed or bloated
- Drinking too much fluid with a meal, which can dilute stomach acid and digestive enzymes: one cup of fluid with a meal is sufficient

All of the above put a strain on your stomach and intestines in their attempt to properly digest and assimilate food. This adds to your stress levels in two ways:

- Directly, through indigestion, bloating, and cramping
- Indirectly, through malabsorption of essential nutrients

If food is not properly digested in your mouth and stomach, much of it will pass through your intestines and will subsequently putrefy and ferment —causing bloating, cramps, and gas.

Resultantly, you will receive only a limited portion of the nutrition potentially available in your food, leading to a subtle form of undernourishment

In addition to reconsidering what you eat to boost your mood, you can decrease stress and anxiety and a probable malabsorption problem by going slowly.

Give yourself adequate time to eat, chewing your food thoroughly, avoid drinking while eating, and not overtaxing your body by eating excessive amounts.

Importantly, prepare ahead. Lack of time, stress, and wanting an instant fix leads many people to fast-food outlets or to forget to eat altogether.

In the next chapter you'll discover the perils of consuming sugar and its derivatives to boost flagging energy levels.

14

SWEET MISERY

If you've been turning to booze to tame your anxiety, or candy and energy drinks consider if it's the taste you're addicted to or whether you're craving sugar? You may be surprised to learn how much sugar is hiding in your alcohol and food (coffee, tea, cola, energy drinks, bread, cereal, salad dressings, processed meat, along with deserts).

You'd probably be blown away to learn that some studies suggest that sugar is 10 times more addictive than cocaine. Cocaine! Not only is sugar in rampant, easy supply, but it's hard to give it up—especially when you're feeling fatigued or stress-eating and searching for comfort.

The result of continually bombarding your body with too much sugar leads to the creation of a chronic dysregulation in sugar metabolism. For some people this dysregulation can lead to excessively high levels of blood sugar, or diabetes.

For an even larger number of people, the problem is just the opposite—periodic drops in blood sugar level *below* normal, a condition known to as *hypoglycemia.*

The symptoms of hypoglycemia tend to manifest when your blood sugar drops below 50 to 60 milligrams per milliliter—or when it plummets very rapidly from higher to lower levels.

Hypoglycemia can also occur simply in *response to stress,* since your body burns up sugar very rapidly under stress.

Note most common symptoms of hypoglycemia include:

- Light-headedness
- Anxiety
- Trembling
- Feelings of unsteadiness or weakness
- Irritability
- Palpitations

These are also some of the symptoms that can accompany a panic attack!

No wonder, that among health conscious people these days, sugar has been somewhat of a dirty word.

Personally, I have always favored the sweeter wines, Riesling, Pinot Gris and Gewurztraminer and others. What I didn't realize was it wasn't the variety of grapes I was attracted to but the higher sugar content.

Until I began researching my book *Mind Your Drink,* I didn't even think about how much sugar I was ingesting, nor was I aware of how many alcohol manufacturers add extra sugar to the mix to keep you hooked.

Two or three glasses of wine can easily contain 3 teaspoons of sugar which is 75 percent of the recommended daily intake for women.

A vodka and cranberry easily hides a whopping seven-and-a-half teaspoons, while a G&T offers little to celebrate at four teaspoons of sugar.

Don't be fooled by companies like Coca-Cola who have developed new sub brands to sell 'healthy' alternatives like Cranberry Juice. I was almost duped until I studied the labels and discovered the differences in sugar content.

Current laws don't compel alcohol companies to disclose what's hidden in booze, including added sugar. Although, higher than recommended levels of sulfites do have to be disclosed. A move in this direction, including sugar content and the addition of harmful artificial sweeteners, must surely be around the corner—especially as obesity, anxiety, and depression levels continue to soar.

A recent report from the Australian Institute of Health and Welfare (AIHW) revealed that Australia has one of the highest rates of obesity in the world —a staggering 63% of adults are overweight and obese. Truly alarming.

Why is obesity an escalating issue? While food, nutrition, and exercise are all culpable nobody seems to be pointing the finger at epidemic levels of sugar-spiked alcohol consumption.

Instead, we're being fed the wrong messages and dispensed the wrong advice.

While beer is said to contain less sugar than other alcoholic alternatives, you only have to survey mens beer-guts to sense something is amiss.

No, over-drinking doesn't make you look sexier.

No wonder my excess weight peeled off and my anxiety subsided when I gave up booze. Plus, once I was free of the sugar cravings (and the with-drawals) it was easier to cut back.

"Sweets, like heroin, enter the body (and hence the brain) very rapidly," says neuroscientist Dr. Candace Pert.

"Sugar is a drug in a very real sense, and we're

addicted to the 'up' feeling we get when our blood-sugar levels soar. This substance directly impacts your molecules of emotion—insulin being the main one. External drugs, internal chemicals, and the emotions— all of these use the exact same pathways and receptors," writes Candace Pert in *Everything You Need to Know to Feel Go(o)d.*

Sugar is a double-edged sword. Falling amounts of sugar can make you feel anxious, panicky, hyperactive, or depressed.

Too much sugar in your diet makes you irritable, keeps you hungry, speeds up the aging process, and spikes irrational cravings.

"The demand for it can override your behavior just as a craving for heroin can, driving you not only to seek more and more sugary foods, but also to engage in behaviors that are associated with blood sugar on the rise. Unlike heroin, however, sugar is legal, plentiful, and cheap, so you're likely to satisfy that drive from the available supply and become hooked without even being aware of it," says Pert.

No wonder giving up alcohol is doubly hard. It's a quick highly addictive double-impact hit and an even quicker descent into sugar-fueled, alcohol-saturated misery if you don't catch on quickly.

A word of caution. Don't even think about swapping your pre-mixes for drinks marketed as 'diet' alternatives. Increasing research warns of the extreme health hazards of Aspartame, an artificial sweetener marketed as Nutrasweet, Equal, and Spoonful (in the UK).

The fact is, however, that your body and brain need glucose—or naturally occurring sugar—in order to operate. Glucose is the fuel your body burns; it provides the energy which sustains your life. Much of this glucose is derived from carbohydrate foods in your diet such as bread, cereal, potatoes, vegetables, fruits, pasta, and so on. The starches in these foods are broken down *gradually* into glucose.

Simple sugars, on the other hand, such as refined white sugar, brown sugar and honey, break down very quickly into glucose. These simple sugars can cause problems because they tend to overload your system with too much sugar too quickly. Our bodies are not equipped to process large amounts of sugar so quickly. Less, really is more, when it comes to consuming sugar. Your mind, body and spirit will love you for it.

For a comprehensive summary of sugar in all its guises I highly recommend Dr. Candace Pert's excellent book, *Everything You Need to Know to Feel Go(o)d.*

DIETARY MODIFICATIONS FOR HYPOGLYCEMIA

- Eliminate as much as possible all types of simple white sugar from your diet. It also includes subtler forms of sugar, such as honey, corn syrup, molasses, and high fructose. Be sure to read the labels on all processed foods to detect various forms of sugar.
- Substitute fruits (other than dried fruits, which are too concentrated in sugar) in pace of sweets. Avoid fruit juices or dilute them 1:1 with water.
- Reduce or eliminate simple starches such as pasta, refined cereals, potato chips, and white bread. Substitute instead complex carbohydrates such as whole grain breads and cereals, vegetables, and brown rice, quinoa or other whole grains.
- Enjoy a complex carbohydrate or protein snack (nuts, whole grain toast and cheese, for example) halfway between meals—around 10:30-11 in the morning and especially around 4-5 in the

afternoon. If you wake early in the morning at 4 or 5, you may find that a small snack will help get you back to sleep for a few well-needed hours. As an alternative to snacks between meals, you can try having four or five small meals per day no more than two to three hours apart. The aim is to maintain steadier blood sugar levels

15

AVOID OVER-STIMULATION

Sometimes the best way to bounce is to eat what you don't want, drink what you don't like, and do what you'd rather avoid.

Knock things like coffee, caffeinated drinks and foods, alcohol, and nicotine off your list (or at least limit your intake).

These trigger the production of the stress-related hormone adrenaline—which increases your heart rate, prompts the liver to release more sugar into your bloodstream, and makes the lungs take in more oxygen.

While these things may give you a short-term high, in the long run, the result is fatigue and low energy levels. This in turn, leads to a vicious cycle of relying on more stimulants to get you through the day.

The impact of excessive coffee and caffeinated drinks has become such a health-hazard, a new disorder, Caffeine Use Disorder, was recently added to the DSM-V—the tool psychologists, psychiatrists, and other mental-health professionals often refer to prior to making their diagnosis.

Are you addicted to caffeine?

If you've experienced these three symptoms within the past year—you may be in trouble:

- You have a persistent desire to give up or cut down on caffeine use, or you've tried to do so unsuccessfully.
- You continue to use caffeine despite knowing it contributes to recurring physical or psychological problems for you (like insomnia, or jitteriness).
- You experience withdrawal symptoms if you don't have your usual amount of caffeine.

Many of my clients notice reduced levels of anxiety, irritability, and depression when they kick the habit. They also report feeling better able to cope with stress, once the coffee habit is culled.

Opt for a natural high. Consider replacing caffeine, alcohol, nicotine and other stimulants with fresh juices, exercise, meditation, or some other activity which makes you feel great and sustains energy. Herbal teas are also healthy caffeine-free alternatives. Try to drink 6-8 glasses (1.7-2 liters) of water a day to boost energy and flush out toxins.

Less artificial stimulation means more natural life-affirming highs.

16

MINDFUL DRINKING

Many people mistakenly believe drinking alcohol will increase their happiness. But alcohol is a depressant and in large quantities is draining on your body and mind.

Alcohol has been found in many studies to significantly reduce serotonin 45 minutes after drinking. The sleep rhythms of people who have drunk alcohol the day before are significantly different from controls groups who didn't drink alcohol but very similar to patients with depression.

Numerous studies suggest that low serotonin is the mechanism behind both depression and anxiety after alcohol consumption.

Experience may have already taught you that too much booze increases anxiety, muddles the mind, ignites aggression, reduces responsiveness, and ultimately depresses.

It's also hard to quit—alcohol is one of the most addictive legal drugs on the planet.

It's also a well-documented neurotoxin—a toxic substance that inhibits, damages, and destroys the tissues of your nervous system.

To improve their mental health many people limit their drinking or consciously decide not to touch a drop. Keeping their resolve often takes extraordinary willpower.

Author and public speaker Deepak Chopra gave up drinking. "I liked it too much," he once said. Steven King, after almost losing his family and destroying his writing career, managed to quit.

Other people like Amy Winehouse devastatingly never made it. At only 27, she died of alcohol poisoning in 2011.

The risk of suicide also increases for stressed people who turn to drink. As I've already discussed, alcohol abuse and excessive drinking is a major cause of anxiety and depression, impairs mental reasoning and critical thinking—increasing the likelihood of making tragic and often impulsive choices.

There is also clear evidence between alcohol consumption and violence and other types of aggressive behavior. Aggressive behavior is also heavily linked to low serotonin levels. Some experts suggest that aggressive behavior after a period of alcohol may be due to alcohol's disrupting effects on serotonin metabolism—as little as two standard drinks can ignite anger.

To better understand why people often become aggressive and violent after drinking alcohol, researchers in Australia used magnetic resonance imaging (MRI) scans to measure blood flow in the brain. They noted that after only two drinks, there were changes in the working of the brain's prefrontal cortex, the part normally involved in tempering a person's aggressive levels.

Risking ruining your relationships, ruining your career, sacrificing your sanity, and in the extreme, taking your life, is a massive price to pay for a mistaken belief that to be happy, or to numb your anxiety or cope with stress you need to drink more booze.

Boost your resilience beautifully by exploring your relationship to drink and approaching it more mindfully. Consider, a period of sobriety. Instead of focusing on what you may be giving up, turn your mind to what you may gain—a better, more energized version of yourself.

The many benefits of reducing your alcohol intake, or not drinking at all, include:

- A stronger ability to focus on your goals and dreams
- Improved confidence and self-esteem
- Increased productivity
- Increased memory, mental performance, and decision-making
- Better control of your emotions
- Sweeter relationships
- Greater intuition and spiritual intelligence
- Authentic happiness

Your body never lies, but many people soldier on, ignoring the obvious warning signs that it's time to scale back their drinking or lose the booze.

- Headaches
- Anxiety
- Depression
- Insomnia
- Aggression
- Blackouts
- Low energy and fatigue
- High blood pressure

...are just a few of many signs that it may be time to control alcohol before it controls you.

It's easy to rationalize these feelings away, but the reality is that your mind, body, and soul are screaming out for liberation.

Have the courage to say 'yes' to pursuing a more energizing alternative.

Your body is a great source of wisdom and counsel —one that is increasingly respected by psychologists and medical professionals. *Somatic Psychology*, a branch of traditional psychotherapy, addresses what for so long was missing in the field of talk therapy.

Soma is a Greek word meaning "the living body" and is grounded in the belief that not only are thought, emotion and bodily experience inextricably linked (creating a *bodymind*), but also that change can be brought about in one domain of experience by mindfully accessing another.

You may consider asking your body next time you feel tempted to drink or feel the first flush of alcohol hit your system, "what does this beer (or whatever you are drinking) want me to know?" This may seem weird, but stick with me!

When I tried this recently, my body told me, "This alcohol makes me feel sick. I don't want it. Don't drink any more of it."

My mind, however, was telling me a different

and conflicting story as it rattled through a range of old stories and false beliefs.

In this case, as in others, I trusted my body barometer.

Very often people don't listen to their body barometers until it's too late and health havoc can set in. Leonardo da Vinci once said that people were more motivated to act by fear than they were by love. I'll let you decide, but whether the joy of health nirvana or the fear of health havoc rules supreme, as long as you heed the call for change you'll always win.

HEALTH NIRVANA

Controlling alcohol consumption or quitting for good has numerous positive benefits. Everything is interconnected but let's try to categorize a few of the health benefits you can expect with sobriety:

Physical Health

- Improved liver function and health
- Better sleep
- Better eating habits
- Younger, healthier looking skin, hair, and nails

- Improved vision and clearer eyes
- Weight loss or healthy weight gain
- Increased energy and vitality
- Strengthened immune system, warding off illness and disease
- Lower blood pressure
- Optimal digestive function

Mental Health

- Increased mental clarity
- Newfound motivation and determination
- Natural resilience
- Boost self-esteem and confidence
- Greater resilience to stress
- Improved memory
- Clarity
- Heightened intuition
- Heightened brain function
- Improved productivity
- Heightened sensory skills—everything looks, feels, tastes, sounds clearer and brighter
- Heightened willpower
- More truthfulness and honesty

- Long and short-term memory improves
- Aversion to negative thinking
- Improvement of coexisting conditions (anxiety, depression, bipolar, etc.)
- A desire to help others

Emotional Health

- Persistent and lasting feelings of joy
- Authentic happiness
- Improved relationships
- Increased joy of looking and feeling healthier and better about yourself
- Increased ability to create lasting, loving relationships
- Improved interactions with people
- Feeling younger
- Feeling empowered, in control and free
- More laughter and spontaneous joy
- Improved general sense of contentment and wellbeing
- Greater self-awareness
- Higher emotional intelligence and ability to self-regulate
- An improved sleep-related benefits

- Increased interest and engagement in new activities, hobbies or learning
- Feelings of freedom, hope, self-worth, and self-empowerment

If alcohol is a known cause for more than 60 different adverse health conditions, I'm betting sobriety is a known cause of more than 60 different positive health conditions—maybe even triple that. But finding data to back me up is hard to find. It seems more money is poured into measuring harm than keeping statistics related to health.

Keep your own stats and set yourself up to succeed. To support and maintain your sobriety, really absorb all the benefits. Enjoy the anticipated positive results of sobriety at the start of your day, in the evening, or whenever you have a spare moment.

When you are sober, be sure to be mindful and really enjoy the results of your efforts. For example, as I write this chapter, notice I'm feeling energized, clear-headed, purposeful, and excited. I have the youthful expectant energy of a child. I feel a sense of self-worth with all that I have achieved today. I think I may take a wee break now, reward myself and go out and play!

I also draw my attention to how much I appreciate and value my improved relationship with my partner and my mother, and I love, love, love that I'm a positive influence on my 26-year-old daughter who has chosen to go alcohol-free and is not only loving it but is positively influencing all her friends. Her anxiety has disappeared and she is glowing.

I have way more self-belief and am both less critical of others and myself, and no longer hyper-sensitive to others barbs and attacks when I don't drink.

Did drinking less alcohol do all that? Not entirely. As I said earlier, controlling alcohol requires a systemic approach and making lifestyle changes both in health behaviors and other factors which I discuss throughout my sobriety books, *Mind Your Drink* and *Your Beautiful Mind.*

Putting the spotlight on the harm alcohol caused me, my family, my loved ones, within my community and the world at large also drives me. Negatives can be positives when seen in the right light and used constructively.

I no longer feel like the booze hag who once wrote this:

"Pretty much four months after I decided to say no to booze, but the little bugger has slipped into my psyche

again. Last night and the night before I had two vodkas and orange—freshly squeezed. 4pm-ish. I watched myself, observed myself. The knowledge that I was tired, weary, that I needed to meditate.

But I wanted that quick fix.

That nice little forgetting of alcohol. But who's paying now? 12:15 A.M. and I'm wide awake. I haven't woken like this in months. I don't feel flash either. Yesterday I was excited about my book Flight of Passion—now I feel like it's crap. It's the depressing booze, my head aches, my throat and chest burns."

Instead, in my journal 'sober me' wrote:

Hello Sunday Morning! I'm so grateful for John's drunkenness last night. It's strengthened my resolve. I want nothing to with the poison of drink—unless it's with a refined meal or a celebration. I've woken up clear-headed, clear-hearted, my energy bright, looking forward to the day.

"When you are full of food and drink an ugly statue sits where your spirit should be." ~ Rumi

Even if people think it's no big deal to drink a glass of wine at dinner it's important to know your body's reaction to alcohol and not just go along with the crowd.

I'd forgotten my assignment on spiritual approaches to the treatment of alcohol addiction. I must revisit it.

A blackbird rustles amongst Autumn leaves. John is at his desk. The door is shut. I walk past the front window. "Would you like an orange juice?"

No, he wouldn't.

His eyes are dead, remorseful—as though regretting his foolishness. His skin is gray, pallid, like that of a dying man.

Rumi is right....an ugly statue sits where his spirit should be.

Even the Romans once ate and drank from a lead cup. *Poison in poison.*

HEALTH HAVOC

When you pollute your body with alcohol, a known carcinogen, and neurotoxin, it's going to play havoc with your health. Big time. Perhaps not today, not tomorrow, but it will happen, and when it does, I doubt you'll be happy about it.

You may even swear and curse your stupidity, as my step-father did when he was diagnosed with terminal lung cancer, "You bloody stupid fool," he said, sadly and stoically accepting his fate when told he had a month to live. Having enjoyed smoking for many years, I know he would have done anything to undo the wrongs of the past.

Alcohol, as I have said, is a known cause for more than 60 different adverse health conditions, listed below are just a few:

PHYSICAL HEALTH

- Carcinogenic—causes cancer in living tissue. Strong links between cancers of the liver, breast, bowel, upper throat, mouth, esophagus and larynx
- Negatively affects brain development in young people
- Depresses your entire nervous system
- Compromises your immune system, making you less resistant to illness and disease
- Interferes with the body's ability to absorb calcium, resulting in bones that are weaker, softer, and more brittle
- Kills cells and disrupts cellular metabolic processes
- Distorts your eyesight, making it difficult to adjust to the differing light and compromising clarity
- Diminishes your ability to distinguish

between sounds and perceive their direction
- Slurs your speech
- Dulls your sense of taste and smell
- Damages the lining of your throat
- Weakens your muscles
- Inhibits the production of white and red blood cells
- Destroys your stomach lining
- Poisons you and can cause death
- Disrupts your sleep cycle, reduces rapid eye movement (REM) sleep, creates insomnia
- Suppresses breathing and can precipitate sleep apnea
- Increases weight or causes unhealthy weight loss
- Strips your body of vital nutrients and causes malnutrition
- Increases the likelihood of indulging in risky, unsafe and unlawful behaviors
- Heightens suicidal thoughts

MENTAL HEALTH

- Causes anxiety and depression and other mental disorders

- Lowers the levels of serotonin in your brain—a chemical that helps to regulate your mood
- Destroys your brain cells
- Increases suicidal tendencies
- Negatively impacts memory
- Causes permanent damage to your brain
- Alters your brain chemistry
- Escalates aggression
- Increases stress levels
- Triggers dormant mental illnesses (bi-polar etc.)
- Disruptions in REM sleep may cause daytime drowsiness, poor concentration, and low mood
- Depletes willpower

EMOTIONAL HEALTH

- Undermines your self-esteem and self-respect
- Depletes your courage, confidence
- Undermines your relationships with your partner, family, and friends
- Contributes to depression
- Reduces self-control
- Increases the difficulty in maintaining

healthy relationships, including with
bosses, co-workers and, clients
- Creates financial strain, leading to more
stress, worry any and anxiety

AND THAT'S JUST a few ways that alcohol can play havoc with your health. The increased risk of developing arthritis, cancer, heart disease, hyperglycemia and hypoglycemia, kidney disease, obesity, nervous disorders, and many psychological disturbances can all be attributed to alcohol abuse. And as you know, acute alcohol poisoning can cause death.

Find out more about short and long-term effects that drinking alcohol has on many different parts of your body here—https://www.alcohol.org.nz/alcohol-its-effects/body-effects.

Your mind and body may seem like separate entities but when you let your body override your craving mind you find a reservoir of unbridled power. Your body barometer never lies, and as we've seen, can save your life by expelling toxins from your system.

When you drink alcohol or feel hung over what

do you notice? How does this differ from times when you feel sober?

If you fall off the wagon and start drinking again don't be too hard on your beautiful self. Practice mindfulness and self-compassion and tune into your body barometer.

How do you feel? Have the headaches, nausea, depression, aggression or anxiety returned again?

Journal your experience as I did to reinforce your awareness and to strengthen your resolve to stop drinking again.

You'll find helpful sobriety journalling tips in my book, *The Sobriety Journal: The Easy Way to Stop Drinking: The Effortless Path to Being Happy, Healthy and Motivated Without Alcohol.*

THE PATH TO SOBRIETY

In my books *Mind Your Drink* and *Your Beautiful Mind,* I break down the path to sobriety in ways you can easily understand and apply to your own life.

Knowledge is power. Ultimately long-term success in winning the war on alcohol can be explained through medical science and psychology— and understanding the psychological warfare tactics of the world's best marketers. You do realize that the booze barons act narcissistically to encourage you to act against your best interests, right?

Understanding alcohol from all angles offers substantive reasons for why it keeps you hooked.

Importantly, what I'd love you to take away from reading this book, and those focused on controlling alcohol is that there is no one path to sobriety. You may or may not be able to go it alone, you may need help, you may need therapy, but regardless of the approach you take, controlling alcohol is a long-term lifestyle change.

Very often, as I've said, it may mean spotlighting and healing the wounds of your past.

In my books *Mind Your Drink* and *Your Beautiful Mind* comedian and former addict Russel Brand shares his story of childhood sexual abuse in his book *Recovery: Freedom From Our Addictions*. In his book, he reinterprets The Twelve Step recovery process and champions the call for abstinence.

Similarly, Duff McKagan, the former bass guitarist of Guns N' Roses and one of the world's greatest rock musicians, shares how he used alcohol to self-medicate his agonizing anxiety. The origin of his pain he says stemmed from being asked to lie to his mother about his father's affairs, their subsequent divorce, and his father's own heavy drinking.

McKagan devised his own program of anxiety

treatment and alcohol recovery. Read the inspiring story of a man who partied so hard he nearly died, in his book *It's So Easy and Other Lies.*

Anne Dowsett Johnson, a journalist and self-described recovering alcoholic, and the daughter of an alcoholic herself, urges us all to wake up to the willful blindness to the damages of drinking in our culture, and explores disturbing trends and false promises peddled by alcohol barons in her book *Drink: The Intimate Relationship Between Women and Alcohol.* For Dowsett, medical intervention through prescribed anti-depressants played an instrumental role in her recovery.

AA's 12-step approach didn't work for stressed entrepreneur Russ Parry. But years of therapy, couple counseling, renewing his faith and a program of recovery offered by his church did—alongside changing his relationship to work. He shares his journey to abstinence in his book, *The Sober Entrepreneur.*

These are just some of the many people and books I have come to admire as I embarked on my own journey to understand why I once drank so much and why I couldn't stop.

For these people, sharing their stories was part of their healing process—that and the desire to pay-it-forward. In my book, *Employ Yourself* from my bestselling *Mid-Life Career Rescue* series, I share how health coach Sheree Clark numbed her anxiety, stress and job blues by over-drinking until she realized booze was never going to be a long-term sustainable solution.

She's sold her business and created a new career as a healthy living coach. She still enjoys a drink—but that since her career change that she couldn't be happier or healthier.

As the former addict and leading neuroscientist Marc Lewis writes in this book, *The Biology of Desire: Why Addiction is Not a Disease,* alcoholism, and addiction "can spring up in anyone's backyard. It attacks our politicians, our entertainers, our relatives, and often ourselves. It's become ubiquitous, expectable, like air pollution and cancer."

Shaming, blaming and naming is not the cure, compassion understanding, and living life on your terms is.

As Lewis also notes, "Many experts highlight the value of empowerment for overcoming addiction. In fact, most former addicts claim that empowerment, not powerlessness, was essential to them, especially in the latter stages of their recovery. Sensitivity to the meaning of empowerment in recovery may be greatest for those who've been disempowered in their social world, including women, minorities, the poor, and those with devastating family histories."

Abusing alcohol is not a disease. It's a coping strategy—one, before reading this book, you may not have been aware of.

As you read this book, you'll reclaim your power and decide whether alcohol has anything positive to contribute to your life at all, or whether you'd be better off putting your money, your energy, your time, your happiness and your health into something, or someone, who's a less abusive lover. Yes, you will decide—it's that simple, and at times, that difficult.

Not everyone battles with booze. Whether you cut back or eliminate alcohol entirely, the choice is ultimately yours. Only you know the benefits alcohol delivers or the success it destroys.

You may enjoy reading my blog post on spiritual approaches to the treatment of alcohol addiction—http://www.cassandragaisford.com/spiritual-approaches-to-the-treatment-of-alcohol-addiction/

If you'd like to experiment with a period of sobriety or you need help to you moderate your drinking, *Mind Your Drink: The Surprising Joy of Sobriety*, available as a paperback and eBook will help.

You can also find a range of books and resources offering help to quit, including alcohol-free alternatives on my website—http://www. cassandragaisford.com/books-and-resources/ control-alcohol/

17

JUST ADD WATER

As blood is to your heart, so water is to your body. Our bodies are machines, designed to run on water and minerals. Because we're made up of 72 percent of water, it's vitally important for every bodily function—especially to your liver.

Insufficient water intake and low consumption of fruit and vegetables can present significant health challenges.

Too much coffee, alcohol, or other diuretics (which increase the amount of water and salt expelled from the body as urine) can also rob your mind and body of energy and vitality.

When you're dehydrated, your thoughts become muddled, anxiety can loom, and you'll feel tired, irritable, unmotivated, and generally lackluster.

The link between water and stress reduction is well documented. All of your organs, especially your brain, needs water to function properly. If you're dehydrated, you're not fueling your body for optimum performance—and that can lead to stress and anxiety. Endurance athletes know this very well.

"Studies have shown that being just half a liter dehydrated can increase your cortisol levels," says Amanda Carlson, RD, director of performance nutrition at Athletes' Performance, a trainer of world-class athletes.

Life is an endurance race. Consider the fact, that the more hydrated your body, mind, and spirit is, the longer you'll be able to sustain the pace.

Cortisol is a stress hormone. Staying well hydrated status can keep your cortisol levels regulated and your stress levels down. When you don't give your body the fluids it needs, you're putting unnecessary stress on it, and it's not going to thank you.

That doesn't mean that drinking plenty of water throughout the day will magically cause your relationship woes, your money problems, your childs' troubles at school, and your deadlines at work to disappear. But if you're already stressed by coping with all of these things, you don't need the additional stress of dehydration to add to your burden.

"You're actually likely to get more dehydrated when you're under stress, because your heart rate is up and you're breathing more heavily, so you're losing fluid," says Renee Melton, MS, RD, LD, director of nutrition for Sensei, a developer of online and mobile weight loss and nutrition programs. "And during times of stress, you're more likely to forget to drink and eat well. Just getting enough fluids helps to keep you at your best during times like these."

BREAK THE ANXIETY CYCLE

Anxiety can cause dehydration, and dehydration can cause anxiety. It's a bullying cycle. You can beat it by building more water consumption into your day. Stress and anxiety can result in many of the same responses as dehydration— increased heart rate, nausea, fatigue, and headaches.

So, if you can remain hydrated you can reduce the magnitude of the physiological responses you have to stressful events and anxiety-inducing situations.

How else do you know if you are dehydrated?

Firstly, are you thirsty? If you are, you're already dehydrated.

Secondly, take a look at the toilet bowl next time you go to the bathroom. If the urine is dark in color and has a pungent smell, you're dehydrated. The darker the urine and the stronger the smell, the more dehydrated you are.

TIPS FOR DRINKING ENOUGH WATER EACH DAY

How can you build more water consumption into your day? Try these tips:

- Carry an insulated sports bottle with you and fill it up periodically.
- Keep a glass of water on your desk at work.
- Keep another glass next to your bed. Many of us wake up dehydrated first thing in the morning.
- Switch one glass of soda or cup of coffee for a glass of water.
- Drink at least eight glasses (in small amounts) of purified water throughout the day. Six glasses all at once isn't good for you!
- Consume more fruits and vegetables—as close to raw as possible

Try to drink 6-8 glasses (1.7-2 liters) of water a day to boost energy and flush out toxins. Sip more water during those high-stress times and remember to reduce or avoid beverages and foods and lifestyle choices that dehydrate you—such as coffee, wine, cigarettes and salty foods.

IMMERSE YOURSELF

In addition to drinking H_2O, many people also find gazing upon or immersing themselves in a body of natural water promotes a positive mindset.

It's no coincidence that most millionaires have houses overlooking water.

I love to bathe in the hot mineral waters at Ngawha Springs in the far north of New Zealand. Local Maori have long known of the therapeutic properties of bathing in its waters. Even if I feel low, I always emerge feeling great, and my energy and health are always instantly restored.

Create more energy and drive by flushing toxins from your body as well as increasing your connection with water. Some simple, but effective strategies include:

- Splash water on your face whenever

you're feeling overwhelmed. Cold water steps up circulation, making you feel invigorated

- Swim in the sea or a lake, or bathe in hot mineral water—either in a natural spring or by adding Epsom Salts (a mineral compound of magnesium and sulfate) to your bath.

18

FOOD ALLERGIES AND ANXIETY

Many people go for years without recognizing that the very foods they crave the most have a subtle but toxic effect on their mood and well-being.

Allergic reactions occur when your body attempts to fight the intrusion of a foreign substance. For some people certain foods and substances create allergic reactions.

These allergies can cause not only classic symptoms such as a runny nose, mucous, but also trigger the following psychological or psychosomatic symptoms:

- Anxiety or panic
- Depression and mood swings
- Dizziness
- Irritability

- Insomnia
- Headaches
- Confusion and disorientation
- Fatigue

Typical foods that can create an allergic response include:

- Alcohol
- Chocolate
- Citrus fruits
- Corn
- Eggs
- Peanuts
- Yeast
- Shellfish
- Soy Products
- Tomatoes
- Gluten/wheat

One of the most telling signs of food allergy is addiction. We often tend to crave and are addicted to the very foods we are allergic to.

To discover whether your food allergies are aggravating your anxiety levels, you may wish to consult your doctor or visit a nutritionist.

One of my clients, a successful financial trader, in his late 30s suddenly started experiencing mood swings, anxiety and depression. He decided to go to a nutritionist who sent samples of his hair away to test for food allergies.

What was uncovered was not only allergies to some foods, but a high degree of aluminum in his body which was traced to his deodorant. Making changes to both his diet and to his hygiene products resulted in a dramatic change to his mental health

Some research suggests that aluminum is so abundant and widely used in modern life that increasing amounts of this toxic metal are stored in our brains and bodies, potentially increasing our risk of anxiety and serious diseases.

Protecting yourself from the toxic effects of aluminum poisoning includes taking care to avoid ingesting it or exposing yourself to it through medications, skin care products and other sources of aluminum contamination.

Here are just a few of many strategies to aid the fight against aluminium poisoning and protect your nervous system.

L-theanine

L-theanine is an amino acid derivative primarily found in tea. It has been reported to promote relaxation, relieve perceptions of stress, and protect the nervous system. One study found L-theanine was effective in alleviating the negative effects of aluminum-induced toxicity.

If you want to take L-theanine, take a 200-mg capsule before bed. If you typically suffer from anxiety or feel highly stressed, you can also try an additional 200 mg of L-theanine during the day for enhanced relaxation without sedation. Reduce your stress and protect your brain simultaneously.

Green tea

Green tea extract contains small amounts of L-theanine, along with other important compounds with medicinal effects and studies have found it also aids in the fight against aluminum poisoning.

Green tea extract and L-theanine used in combination was found to also reverse aluminum toxicity and treat cognitive impairment even better.

In one recent randomized, double-blind, placebo-controlled study, 91 patients with mild cognitive impairment took 1,680 mg per day of a combination of L-theanine and green tea extract for 16 weeks.

The combination treatment led to improvements in memory and selective attention. Brain theta waves, an indicator of cognitive alertness, were increased significantly for three hours.

Are you allergic to meat? Perhaps your 'allergy' stems from a personal conviction that eating meat doesn't feel right to you. Before we move from away from dietary contributors to stress, I also wanted to share the recent experience of a client of mine who came for counseling.

A key component of John's anxiety and depression stemmed from childhood trauma, and these, along with problems he was experiencing in his relationship, led to him to seek counseling.

During our sessions he also went to visit his doctor who, after taking some blood tests, highlighted John's deficiency of vitamin B12.

Vitamin B12 has a major influence on the healthy functioning of neurons and also on the ability of the bone marrow to make red blood cells.

The effects of B12 deficiency are widespread, and can contribute to almost any psychiatric symptom-from anxiety, and panic to depression and hallucinations.

Key sources of B12 vitamins for anxiety are found in grass-fed beef (especially beef liver), lamb, venison, eggs and yogurt—none of which he consumed. John was a vegan and had been for many years.

It had never occurred to him that his diet was contributing to his anxiety levels. His doctor topped his levels of B12 with an injection and supplements.

Again, as I highlight throughout *The Anxiety Cure,* reducing anxiety often involves a multi-faceted, a multi-disciplinary approach.

Dietary changes alone are seldom the only cure and do not always create lasting results.

19

FEND OFF PANIC ATTACKS

Panic attacks involve a triggering of the fight-or-flight response that helps us react quickly to danger. However, people who experience panic attacks are not necessarily in any danger. A panic attack can arrive with no warning, and no imminent threat.

Experts don't know what causes panic attacks. Stressful life events or heredity may play a role in certain cases (people with close relatives who have suffered an attack have four times the risk). Other theories involve an imbalance of chemicals in the brain, greater sensitivity in brain circuits that process feelings of fear, or an over-reaction to changes in carbon dioxide levels. Professional assessment should be considered for frequent attacks.

HOW TO RECOGNISE PANIC ATTACK SYMPTOMS

A panic attack may occur without any warning and usually passes within a few minutes. It involves intense feeling of extreme fear, and involves at least four of the following symptoms:

- A feeling of imminent catastrophe or doom, or a need to escape; fear of "going crazy" or dying; feelings of un-reality or being detached from oneself
- Pounding heart or chest pain
- Trembling, sweating and shaking
- Difficulty breathing or shortness of breath
- Flushing, chills, or hot flashes
- Numbness or tingling sensations
- Dizziness or lightheadedness; nausea

As you discovered in the chapter, *Sweet Misery*, for some people panic reactions may actually be caused by hypoglycemia.

When suffering a panic attack, it's important to self-soothe. Help yourself by reminding yourself that you're not dying or losing your mind. Take slow deep breaths, and progressively tighten and relax muscles from your toes to your shoulders and arms to release tension.

Tell yourself that you'll feel better in a few moments—because you absolutely will.

Often people recover from panic simply by having something to eat. As their blood sugar rises their body restores to balance and they feel better.

However, the majority of people with panic disorder or other anxiety-related disorders, such as agoraphobia, find that their panic reactions do not necessarily correlate with bouts of low blood sugar.

Again, boosting your resilience, priming your body, mind and spirit for optimum health will help.

As you'll discover in the next chapter, many people find that adopting a daily Yoga practice tames anxiety and delivers many additional benefits.

YOGA

Yoga, relaxation, and mindfulness practices work behind-the-scenes to help lower the stress hormone cortisol.

Just two 90-minute classes a week is enough to notice an improved stress response, even in those who report being highly distressed, according to research on yoga and meditation coming out of Germany. Study participants noted a decrease in stress, anxiety, and depression.

I came across the following quote, source unknown, and it seems to summarize the key benefits of yoga—flexibility...in body, mind, and spirit: "Blessed are the flexible, for they shall not be bent out of shape."

Yoga classes don't have to be difficult. They can vary from gentle and soothing to strenuous and challenging; the choice of style tends to be based on personal preference and physical ability.

Hatha yoga is the most common type of yoga practiced in the United States and combines three elements: physical poses, called *asanas*; controlled breathing practiced in conjunction with asanas; and a short period of deep relaxation or meditation.

"Available reviews of a wide range of yoga practices suggest they can reduce the impact of exaggerated stress responses and may be helpful for both anxiety and depression. In this respect, yoga functions like other self-soothing techniques, such as meditation, relaxation, exercise, or even socializing with friends," says an article posted by Harvard Medical School.

"By reducing perceived stress and anxiety, yoga appears to modulate stress response systems. This, in turn, decreases physiological arousal — for example, reducing the heart rate, lowering blood pressure, and easing respiration. There is also evidence that yoga practices help increase heart rate variability, an indicator of the body's ability to respond to stress more flexibly."

Researchers at the Walter Reed Army Medical Center in Washington, D.C., are offering a yogic method of deep relaxation to veterans returning from combat in Iraq and Afghanistan. Dr. Kristie

Gore, a psychologist at Walter Reed, says the military hopes that yoga-based treatments will be more acceptable to the soldiers and less stigmatizing than traditional psychotherapy. The center now uses yoga and yogic relaxation in post-deployment PTSD awareness courses and plans to conduct a controlled trial of their effectiveness in the future.

Here are a few of the many reported benefits of yoga:

- Improvements in perceived stress, depression, anxiety, energy, fatigue, and well-being
- Reduced tension, anger, and hostility
- Reduced headaches and back pain
- Improved sleep quality
- Improved breathing and deeper relaxation

"Samskara saksat karanat purvajati jnanam. Through sustained focus and meditation on our patterns, habits, and conditioning, we gain knowledge and understanding of our past and how we can change the patterns that aren't serving us to live more freely and fully." ~ Yoga Sutra III.

21

TAKE A DEEP BREATH

In a state of joy and relaxation, you breathe in a deep circular pattern, your heart comes into coherence, and you begin to produce alpha brain waves, giving you access to your own natural tranquillizers and antidepressants.

But under stress your breathing is reversed. Instead of breathing slowly and deeply your breathing tends to become shallower and more rapid.

Breathing is part of your autonomic nervous system (ANS)—the system is in charge of essential bodily processes that you don't need to put any thought into, such as: how fast you breathe, blood pressure, and overall body temperature.

During times of extreme stress, you can forget to breathe at all. You may even hyperventilate—

breathing in an abnormally rapid, deep, or shallow pattern. You will exhale too much carbon dioxide, and as the level of carbon dioxide in the blood drops, the blood vessels narrow, allowing less blood to circulate. If too little blood reaches your brain, you'll become dizzy and may faint.

Calcium in the blood also decreases, causing some muscles and nerves to twitch. The twitching may result in a tingling or stabbing sensation near your mouth or in your chest. These symptoms include a tight feeling in the chest, as though your lungs cannot receive enough air.

This sensation leads to faster and deeper breathing. Your heart may begin to pound, and your pulse rate may rise.

Experiencing these symptoms will increase anxiety in some people, which can make the condition worse—and may even lead to panic attacks.

The ANS has two main components: the sympathetic and parasympathetic divisions. Each component is responsible for different bodily functions.

The sympathetic usually gets these processes going, it also controls your instinctive fight-flight response. The parasympathetic is in charge of everyday processes and stops them from happening.

So even though most ANS functions are automatic and involuntary, you can control some of your ANS processes by doing deep breathing exercises.

Taking deep breaths can help you voluntarily regulate your ANS, which can have many benefits —especially by lowering your heart rate, regulating blood pressure, and helping you relax, all of which help decrease how much of the stress hormone cortisol is released into your body.

If you feel an anxiety attack coming, your breathing starts to race, or you have forgotten how to breathe, try the exercise below:

Breathe in deeply through your nose for a count of four—draw the air up from your belly as though you are inhaling through a straw. You should experience the air moving through your nostrils into your stomach, making your belly expand. During this type of breathing, make sure your stomach is moving outward while your chest remains relatively still.

Now exhale—slowing for a count of eight. You may find it helpful to purse your lips (as if you're about to drink through a straw), press gently on your stomach, and exhale slowly for about two seconds.

Repeat several times for optimal results.

. . .

Numbered breathing

Numbered breathing is another great strategy for gaining control over your breathing patterns and inducing a state of calm. Here's how you can do it:

- Stand up straight and close your eyes
- Inhale deeply until you can't take in anymore air
- Exhale until your lungs have been emptied of all air
- Keep your eyes closed. Now, inhale again while picturing the number 1 in your mind
- Keep the air in your lungs for a few seconds, then exhale it all out
- Inhale again while picturing the number 2.
- Hold your breath while counting silently to 3, then let it all out again
- Repeat these steps until you've reached 10. Feel free to count higher if you want

Notice how quickly your body and mind relaxes. Try this anywhere, anytime you notice feelings of stress, anxiety, or panic returning, and beat the stress response.

Or tap into a meditation or yoga class for enhanced breathing practice with the added benefit of a mind-body makeover.

2 2

GET OUTSIDE

When you're suffering from low mood or feeling anxious very often a lack of outside time is the culprit.

You're like a flower—you need at least 20 minutes of sunlight every day just to make your hormones work effectively and enable you to blossom to your fullest potential.

To feel and behave normally you need to be exposed to full-spectrum daylight on a regular basis. Medical research suggests some people need as much as two hours a day of sunlight to avoid Seasonal Affective Disorder.

Combine outside time with exercise like walking and not only will you get the light you need, but you'll also recharge your batteries.

Walking outside can also help you gain a new

perspective on a troubling situation. When you go outside and take a walk, you increase the electrical activity in your brain, and you breathe negative ions and see in three dimensions.

All this helps you see with fresh eyes the things which are worrying you. Often you'll find that things are not as bad as they first appear, or discover a relatively simple solution.

Monitor how much time you spend indoors. Bounce away from habits like spending too many hours inside in front of two-dimensional computer monitors and TV screens, and then topping off a 12-hour day at work by trying to read yourself to sleep on your Kindle. These are all two-dimensional visual activities, which seldom spark joy.

Let mother earth, the sea and the infinite sky boost your mood. Get outside and allow the sun and outside energy to lift your spirits. Schedule regular fresh air time. Improve your breathing and take a brisk walk to increase your oxygen levels.

23

TAP YOUR WAY TO HAPPINESS

Many people have successfully reduced anxiety by tapping their way to health. Also referred to as psychological acupressure, tapping is a key tool used in the Emotional Freedom Technique (EFT).

EFT tapping is an alternative acupressure therapy treatment used to restore balance to your body's disrupted energy. It's been an authorized treatment for war veterans with PTSD, and medical research has also demonstrated EFT's benefits in the successful treatment of anxiety, depression, physical pain, and insomnia.

According to its creator and EFT founder an imbalance in your energy is the cause of all negative emotions and pain.

People who use this technique believe tapping

key meridian points, or energy hotspots on your body can restore harmony and balance.

It's also believed that repairing this energy imbalance can relieve symptoms which a traumatic episode, negative experience, or toxic emotion may have caused.

Based on Chinese medicine, meridian points are viewed as areas within the body that energy flows through. These pathways help balance energy flow to maintain your health. Toxic emotions and experiences are said to create energy blocks and lead to stagnant energy. This imbalance can influence mental and physical disease or sickness.

While acupuncture uses fingers to apply pressure to these energy points, EFT uses fingertip tapping to apply pressure.

Proponents say the tapping helps you access your body's energy centers and send signals to the part of the brain that controls stress and anxiety.

THE EFT TAPPING SEQUENCE

The EFT tapping sequence employs the methodic tapping on the ends of nine meridian points.

There are 12 major meridians that mirror each side of the body and correspond to an internal organ. However, EFT mainly focuses on these nine:

- karate chop (KC): small
  intestine meridian
- top of head (TH): governing vessel
- eyebrow (EB): bladder meridian
- side of the eye (SE): gallbladder meridian
- under the eye (UE): stomach meridian
- under the nose (UN): governing vessel
- chin (Ch): central vessel
- beginning of the collarbone (CB): kidney
  meridian
- under the arm (UA): spleen meridian

Begin by tapping the karate chop point while simultaneously reciting your setup phrase three times. The setup phrase involves naming the issue causing you anxiety or worry, and affirming that you love and accept yourself anyway—this unconditional self-acceptable removes blame and guilt, which only increases anxiety.

For example, "Even though I'm feeling anxious and worried about my credit card debt, I deeply and completely love and accept myself."

Then, tap each following point seven times, moving down the body in this ascending order:

- eyebrow
- side of the eye
- under the eye

- under the nose
- chin
- beginning of the collarbone
- under the arm

After tapping the underarm point, finish the sequence at the top of the head point.

While tapping the ascending points, recite a reminder phrase to maintain focus on your problem area. If your setup phrase is, "Even though I'm sad my mother is sick, I deeply and completely love and accept myself," your reminder phrase can be, "The sadness I feel that my mother is sick." Recite this phrase at each tapping point. Repeat this sequence two or three times.

At the end of your sequence, rate your intensity level on a scale from 0 to 10. Compare your results with your initial intensity level. If you haven't reached 0, repeat this process until you do.

If reading about how to tap successfully is doing your head in, check out the work of Brad Yates who shares a wonderful way to self-help your way from anxiety to self-love in his YouTube videos. You can check out one of many here —https://youtu.be/K6kq9N9Yp6E.

Yates is not a licensed therapist and therefore cannot officially 'treat' anxiety but I have shared his videos with many of my clients and also used his technique myself and the results have been life-changing.

DOES EFT TAPPING WORK?

EFT has been used to effectively treat war veterans and active military personnel with PTSD. In a 2013 study, researchers studied the impact of EFT tapping on veterans with PTSD against those receiving standard care.

Within a month, participants receiving EFT coaching sessions had significantly reduced their psychological stress. In addition, more than half of the EFT test group no longer fit the criteria for PTSD.

There are also some success stories from people with anxiety using EFT tapping as an alternative treatment.

A 2016 review compared the effectiveness of using EFT tapping over standard care options for anxiety symptoms. The study concluded there was a significant decrease in anxiety scores compared to participants receiving other care.

As I shared in my book, *Mid-Life Career Rescue: Employ Yourself*, many people have successfully used tapping to slay their fear demons and empower their lives.

Jenny Clift, for example, is a professional freelance violinist who currently lives in Madrid, Spain. She is a gifted musician and a natural story-teller. In her book *The Music Inside*, shares her story of reinvention and how she successfully slayed her fear demons and reclaimed her life.

Jenny's book is a powerful memoir of healing. Through books (bibliotherapy!), tapping and the Emotional Freedom Technique, Law of Attraction principals, Esther Hicks and spiritual channeling, therapy and journaling—and music of course—Jenny courageously, honestly and passionately shares her journey back to her fearless, anxiety-free and authentic creative self.

"Most people die with their music still locked up inside them," Benjamin Disraeli once said. This quote was a potent wake-up call to Jenny. She had traded in her dreams of being a concert violinist for the 'safety' of teaching children to play violin.

"Yes, I did know what I wanted to do, but I didn't know how to turn that passion into a living. It felt impossible and I had a laundry list of reasons why I couldn't be a professional violinist:

I'm too old

I'm not good enough

I started too late

It's just not 'me'

How can I rock the boat?

I don't have anyone to help me

How can I walk away from a perfectly good job with the economic situation the way it is now?

I really didn't see that it was possible for me at this stage, but at the same time, that life was eating me up from the inside. Looking back, I realize that's exactly what had to happen–I needed a change from the inside out.

And so I did make it happen. Not overnight. But I started the process that has led me to where I am now—a new place of possibility and job satisfaction. A place where I know that I am doing the right thing at last.

Along the way I have met many new people and have made friends and found mentors who have supported, guided, and taught me many things throughout my journey. I have even improved the relationships I already had, as I have become a happier, more confident, and fulfilled person."

Jenny's book *The Music Inside*, spoke to me on so many levels. As a holistic therapist, counselor and recovering perfectionist I fully endorse the techniques Jenny shares in her book to work on your inner self in order to make outer changes that really work.

I encourage, as Jenny does, anyone who feels trapped in a life or career they no longer want, and for whom unhelpful beliefs and past hurt and saboteurs may be keeping them stuck, to be open-minded and experiment with both cognitive and spiritual approaches to healing.

I also recommend you pick up your body and move to a less stressful and more mood-enhancing career. You'll find plenty of help to do just that in my best-selling series, *Mid-Life Career Rescue: How to Confidently Leave a Job You Hate, and Start Living a Life you Love, Before It's Too Late.*

Perhaps it's not a career change you need but more rest you need—learn more in the chapter which follows.

24

REST

When your stress levels are high and you get depressed, angry, tense, and lethargic or begin to experience tension headaches etc., that should be a very simple biofeedback signal that you need to stop, re-evaluate your choices and take some time out.

Sometimes this can be easier said than done. In our overachiever, overstimulated society, where many people spend more hours every week with their eyes riveted to their iPhone, instead of spending quality time on their own or with family and friends, the whole concept of stopping and resting to restore ourselves seems unusual. But resting to replenish is essential to our well-being.

We're pushing ourselves all day long with energy that we don't have. The most common complaint people consult their doctor for is fatigue.

Research conducted by a company helping people suffering from adrenal fatigue claims that 80% of people don't have as much energy as they'd like to have.

"It's because we're pushing and using caffeine, sugar and energy drinks and nicotine and stress for energy rather than running on our own energy."

Long-term stress and long-term cortisol will literally alter a person's hormonal profile.

Rest allows the adrenal glands to restore, enabling cortisol levels to return to normal. Long-term stress and long-term cortisol overload can lead to adrenal fatigue and burn-out, altering your hormonal profile, and making it more difficult to return to the real, inspired, happy and creative you.

Give yourself permission to take time every day and every week to have fun, rest your mind and rest your body.

25

MASSAGE

One of my favorite ways to rest is to go for a massage. But, so many people mistakenly think massage is an indulgence rather than a health-behavior.

Some of the many benefits of massage include reduced stress and higher levels of neuroendocrine and immune functioning—which means better hormonal balance and more immunity to disease and illness.

Some studies also suggest that a one-hour massage results in benefits equivalent to a 6-hour sleep.

Sounds good to me, especially when I'm feeling fatigued.

If getting naked isn't your thing, consider an

energy healing treatment with a trained Reiki practitioner.

Reiki is a Japanese word. Rei means *universal transcendental spirit* and Ki stands for *life energy*. Hence, the word carries the sense of universal life energy. Many scientific minds, as well as sage healers, have believed throughout the years that the universe is filled with this invisible life energy, and that the life and health of all living beings is sustained by it.

Increasing evidence suggests that there does exist a superior *intelligent force* which contains all creation and out of which all life arises. The energy of this force pervades all things and this is the energy that flows through our hands in concentrated form when we treat with Reiki.

Reiki healing is the ancient art of "hands on healing" and offers a natural and holistic approach to mental, emotional, physical, and spiritual wellbeing.

You don't have to believe in any religion or be particularly spiritual to benefit from Reiki. It's an inclusive, non-religious form of healing and safe for everyone.

When I was experiencing a huge period of stress, I gained so much immediate benefit from my Reiki treatments that I decided to learn this beautiful healing technique. Recently in Bali, I completed my master level training.

You don't have to be Reiki-trained to live by the principles developed by Reiki founder Dr. Mikao Usui: "Just for today do not worry. Just for today do not anger. Honor your parents, teachers and elders. Earn your living honestly. Show gratitude to everything."

Put more fuel in your tank and give yourself the gift of a therapeutic massage or Reiki treatment.

26

TAME YOUR EMAIL MONSTER

Are you suffering from information obesity? Subconsciously, are all your unanswered emails sending your stress levels soaring? Or have text messages become the source of your anxiety?

Email overload is frustrating—and sometimes terrifying. An over-crowded inbox is distracting and will divert your attention from what is important if you don't take charge and do something about it. Your inbox can also house infectious contact from toxic people.

Email, or as my partner calls it, the Email Monster, is the source of many people's anxiety.

Remember that anxiety feeds off fear, uncertainty, overwhelm, and overload. It also loves to distract you from doing the things you enjoy—

burying you in a pyre of often meaningless distractions.

In the last few years, I've also noticed a level of toxicity creeping into emails. Some people are discourteous, and in some instances downright rude and inconsiderate. People rant and vent and type things they might not otherwise have had the courage or lack of manners to say in person.

I'm sure, rather than cowering behind their phone or computer and firing off emails if people stood face-to-face with someone before sending their tirade they wouldn't feel so empowered and emboldened.

The rise in bullying has also led to a whole new malaise—cyberbullying.

Research by Swansea University in 2018, cites that children and young people under 25 who are victims of cyberbullying are more than twice as likely to self-harm and enact suicidal behavior.

The findings also suggest that the perpetrators themselves are at higher risk of experiencing these same suicidal thoughts and behaviors. It's worth remembering that it's the sick who vomit over others, so don't ever take it personally. This is easier said than done.

I've experienced a few toxic battles provoked by others, and there's nothing that spikes my anxiety than the thought of opening my email. It's hard to escape and the scathing words do tend to linger.

Some people clients and customers also send incessant demands, often during the oddest of hours, that they might not request if sending an email were not so spontaneous and instantaneous. Some emails are also lengthy and often arduous to read.

I've also worked with clients, who rather than have honest and frank conversations with each other send emails and texts—corroding their communication with all the mixed messages words not spoken convey.

My partner Laurie feels anxious if he ends his day with one email remaining in his inbox. He receives over 1200 emails a week, and many of his tasks are deadline driven. He manages his anxiety by slaying the Email Monster. He doesn't subscribe to erroneous marketing campaigns promising the golden elixir that will cure us all. Nor does he subscribe to marketing campaigns offering some redundant e-book he would never have time to read and does not care for.

Me? I'm an email hoarder or was. It's stressful and anxiety-producing running my eye over old emails.

This year it's time for the old ways to die.

Before writing this book I was storing over three thousand emails!

It was liberating to press delete. You may gasp in horror at this strategy. But I thought, 'will it really matter, six months from now?' If it does, I'm sure the sender will email me again.

My partner, who I consider to be the king of email efficiency, says you have four choices: answer, unsubscribe, file—out of your inbox and into a 'to answer' file—delete.

"If I don't answer within the timeframe that I feel intuitively is acceptable," he says about his parking strategy, "I go back and delete it. Clearly, it wasn't as important as I first thought."

Consider, simply picking up the phone, or, if you can meet in person, and deal with the issues in the old-fashioned way. It's a myth to think that emails always lead to greater efficiencies.

Be on guard for the Email Monster's equally insidious brother, "Text Dragon." With the advent of voice activation software, I've noticed a lot of people sending lengthy texts. In addition, many people are leaving voice messages on their phones saying, "I don't pick up my messages, if you can't reach me, text instead."

Considerable bullying and abusive behavior, spiking not just anxiety, but also suicidal thoughts and behavior, is being triggered not just by email but text messages too.

Cyber-bullies and those they bully don't just exist with the young, naïve, or immature. In 2019, New Zealand Police began investigating a 'you deserve to die' text sent by one Minister of Parliament to another Minister. Hardly, model leadership behavior.

The recipient received the text well before being sectioned to a mental institution months later, but said in an interview that he re-read the text that day and after texting the MP to say she was going to get her wish, he ended up contemplating suicide.

The text was sent at 1:19am on a Saturday morning—making it even more abusive.

"It was my children that actively stopped me from going through with hurting myself," he told Newshub. "I was just lucky there were people looking for me and lucky that I thought about my little girl's happy face - and not wanting to crush that."

The text message is potentially a breach of the Harmful Digital Communications Act, passed under the then National Government in response to cyberbullying. The law regulated digital communications, including text messages, making it illegal to urge someone to self-harm.

Become skilled with how to block contact from malicious people, and become affirmed with new legislation which offers some protection. Be the change you want to see. Cut down on your digital communication and get real—if you wouldn't say it in person, don't text or email.

If you are ever the target of bullying or abusive behavior seek help and know your rights. Don't horde abusive messages. Slay the Text Dragon and Email Monster and put them firmly in their place.

Think how great it will be with hardly any messages in your inbox. This is how to manage email overload or cyberbullies and reclaim your life!

27

YOUR BEAUTIFUL MIND

When you feel love, joy, gratitude, awe, curiosity, bliss, playfulness, ease, creativity, compassion, growth, or appreciation, you're in your beautiful mind.

Your beautiful mind is in a stream of transcendence and flow. Your spirit and your heart are aligned, and your best self comes alive. Nothing feels like a hassle, everything feels peaceful. You feel no fear or frustration. You're in harmony with your true essence.

Your Suffering Mind

When you're feeling stressed out, worried, frustrated, angry, anxious, depressed, irritable, overwhelmed, resentful, or fearful, your suffering mind has taken control.

Negative feelings and emotions become the norm, even if you'd prefer they weren't.

As I wrote at the beginning of this book, his Holiness the Dalai Lama reminds us, "Nothing beautiful in the end comes without a measure of some pain, some frustration, some suffering."

Reframe your uglies. Take back control, find and prioritize the beauties—the things that spark joy, that give you pleasure and bring deep satisfaction to your mind, body, and soul.

These may be sensory delights, like the smell of fresh coffee, or freshly cut grass, or a whiff of your favorite perfume. Perhaps a stunning photo or a painting sparks joy, or a fabulous piece of architecture. Or, the vivid blue of a summer sky.

Look for the beauty within things you may associate with ugliness. Acknowledge any pain, frustration and suffering as a rite of passage and find beauty in life to reclaim an anxiety-free life.

TAKE RESPONSIBILITY

Whatever is going on in your life you must take personal responsibility. You may not be able to change your circumstances. However, changing yourself is something you can control.

It can take courage to take ownership of your health, happiness, and success. Taking responsibility can mean ending years of blaming others.

Taking responsibility is the ultimate of freedoms. The freedom to be yourself and to choose what happens to you. Coco Chanel once said that she didn't want to weigh more heavily on a man than a bird. She fought for her independence, and created an enduring fortune in the process.

But it's not just about the money. People who take complete responsibility for their lives often experience profound joy and the confidence and added security of knowing they are in the driving seat.

They are able to make wise choices because they know they have ultimate responsibility for those choices and can control how they react to setbacks.

If blaming others or making excuses plays repeatedly in your mind, you are shifting **responsibility** for your decisions and life to others. It's time for some tough and compassionate self-love.

- Eliminate blame, eliminate excuses.
- Commit to an excuse-free diet. Take one hundred percent responsibility for your actions, your thoughts, and your goals. Monitor and be a guard for your words, thoughts and actions.
- Spend time thinking about, and taking action towards your goals, dreams, and desires. Become audaciously inspired and empowered by your visions of success.
- Live every day as if what you do matters —because it does. Every choice you make; every action you take—matters. Your choices matter to you and to the life you live.

- Bounce higher—create your best life by taking back control.

29

ELEVATE YOUR ENERGY

Everything is energy, and energy is everything. Without it you have nothing. But you don't want sad, bad, defeatist energy—that won't help at all.

Passion, joy, and love are the highest vibrations you can feel. They're the rocket-fuel feelings that will catapult you to success.

"The two most inspiring life forces are anger and joy," singer-songwriter Alanis Morissette once said. "I could write 6 zillion songs about these two feelings alone."

As you'll discover in my earlier book, *Find Your Passion and Purpose: Four Easy Steps to Discover a Job You Want and Live the Life You Love*, and in other books in this series, anger can be a constructive force for positive change.

But the more moments you spend being happy

and joyful, and allowing yourself and your work to be infused with this positive energy, the closer you are to being the God-force of all life. You create a natural antidote to anxiety, and you evoke the power of the laws of attraction and abundance, and you attract prosperity.

"If you will live your life in such a manner—that everything you pursue is to make yourself happy— you will live your life to its grandest destiny," writes Ramtha in *The White Book.*

"Joy begets joy, for when you accept the joy that is pressed to you, that joy heightens the joy of your tomorrows and opens you up for ever greater receivership."

Co-creating with joy, passion, Spirit, and love, and creating and maintaining a positive mindset are essential ingredients in raising your productive energy.

Don't worry if you don't know what makes you happy or feel joyful or you haven't figured out where your passions lie. You'll find plenty of help in my other books.

What matters now is that you begin with the end in mind and make a commitment to only invest in things that make you feel good and create positive vibrations.

This may require doing some inner work, increasing your self-awareness and committing to further personal development. It may mean regularly checking in and monitoring your calibration. Or it may involve some tough action.

Many successful people choose to walk away from soul-sucking jobs and relationships to elevate their energy. Paulo Coelho, Isabel Allende, J.K Rowling, Nora Roberts, James Patterson, and Jessie Burton, for example, may not have read Ramtha's sage words which I have quoted below, but they found success by pursuing the love, joy, and purpose they discovered when following their passion.

Importantly, in the process of following their bliss, they all rekindled a deep love for themselves.

"There is no greater purpose in life than to live for the love and fulfillment of self, and that can only be achieved by participating in this life and doing those things which bring you happiness regardless of what they are, for who shall say it is wrong or that it is not good for you?" writes Ramtha in *The White Book*.

What daily practices, routines, or habits fill you with joy? Notice the times you feel marvelous. What soul-sucking jobs, relationships, or situations depress your energy? How can you manifest feel-good vibrations? Develop a plan to restore positivity to your daily diet.

30

SUMMARY OF HOLISTIC STRATEGIES

Throughout this book you've discovered ways to overcome anxiety, build resilience and find joy by increasing your ability to cope. Regular exercise, good diet, relaxation exercises, and rest are a few of the many techniques we've covered.

Listed below are some helpful reminders of some of the many holistic coping strategies we've explored or touched on that you can call upon during times of current or anticipated need. Some of those listed below will be covered in other books in *The Anxiety Cure* series.

PHYSICAL

• Learn to listen to your body

- Adequate exercise
- Getting outside
- Physical touch/massage
- Muscle relaxation
- Sleep
- Warmth
- Relaxation breathing
- A healthy diet, i.e. reducing stimulants (coffee, nicotine, sugar etc.), increasing water, and eating organic non-processed foods, watching for allergies
- Yoga
- Tapping.

BEHAVIORAL

- Balanced lifestyle
- Support groups / counseling
- Sharing with friends and family
- Humor
- New interests / activities
- Hobbies
- Socializing
- Entertaining
- Taking time out
- Music / dancing / singing/ creative expression

- Meditating
- Yoga
- Being proactive and taking control of the situation
- Change careers
- Reducing or eliminating alcohol consumption
- Making time to do nothing at all.

COGNITIVE / PERCEPTUAL (THINKING)

- Rational thinking techniques to help change the way you interpret the stressful situation
- Positive thinking/cultivating optimism
- Self-assertion training
- Personal development
- Building self-esteem
- Realistic goal planning
- Time management
- Learning to say "No"
- Priority clarification
- Reflection
- Mindfulness
- Acceptance
- Hypnosis.

EMOTIONAL

- Releasing emotions and expressing feelings (laugh, talk, cry, write in a journal, paint etc.)
- Learning how to "switch off"
- Taking time out
- Solitude and space
- Intimacy
- Counseling and support
- Challenging your emotional reactions to situations
- Passion/Joy.

SOCIAL

- Scheduling time to spend with important people in your life
- Making plans with friends, family and loved ones in advance
- Sharing your experiences of stress with certain people in your life, especially letting them know the ways that stress has been affecting you, so they understand
- Practicing assertive communication

within your significant relationships to decrease conflicts, while also continuing to find ways to show people around you that they are important.

SPIRITUAL

- Prayer and meditation—scheduling regular time
- Helping others (talking, writing, supporting)
- Reiki and other energy healing techniques
- Talking with a spiritual confidant or leader to explain any spiritual issues or doubts that you may have encountered
- Forgiveness (of self or others)
- Compassion / loving kindness
- Continuing to read and learn about your faith, belief or value system
- Connecting with others who share your beliefs

31

YOUR PLAN TO BUILD
RESILIENCE

Reflect back on the strategies and tools you've discovered in this book. Complete the following exercise to create your personal action plan for beating anxiety, managing stress and building resilience:

Personal Action Plan for Beating Anxiety and Building Resilience

- Factors in your work and life that are causing you the greatest anxiety are:

- The four coping strategies which you know work for you in dealing with anxiety and stress are:

- Your no-excuses strategy to make a commitment to put one or more of these strategies into practice at least once a day is:

- The positive phrase you will use to help change your level of anxiety and stress is:

- Put this phrase where you can see it and say it to yourself when you start to feel stressed.

Complete the following:

I shall stop doing:

I shall do less:

I shall do more:

I shall start to do:

EXCERPT: MID-LIFE
CAREER RESCUE
(EMPLOY YOURSELF)

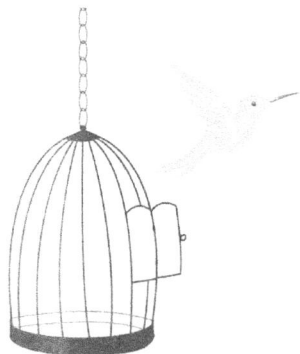

CHOOSE AND GROW YOUR OWN BUSINESS WITH CONFIDENCE

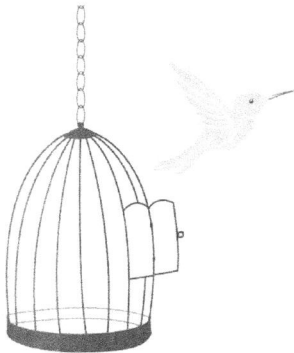

You don't always need buckets of money, or the courage of a lion, to start your own business. Plenty of successful entrepreneurs have started their businesses on a shoe-string budget and launched new careers while combining salaried employment. Many have felt the fear and launched their business anyway.

I was in my mid-30's, a single parent, holding down a steady job, when I started my first business, Worklife Solutions. I was worried and fearful that I'd fail, but I did it anyway. It's one of the most creative, joyful endeavors I've ever done.

Since then I've created many more businesses and helped people all over the globe become successfully self-employed. Like some of the people who share their stories in this book, and other budding entrepreneurs who've taken a strategic route to finance their businesses.

When I first started out in business over a decade ago, I thought about all the people I knew, or had read about, that were successful in their own business. What I found then, still applies today. The list below is what they have in common. As you read this list think how many strategies could apply to you:

They were doing something they love; their passion drove them.

Making money was not their sole motivation. Their businesses grew from a desire to serve others; they were not trying to force something on others or to make a killer sale. Instead, they wanted to make a positive difference and create something of value. They didn't badger people into buying their goods or service.

1. **They cared about whether or not they could help a prospective client.** If they could, great. If not, they were either quietly persistent until they were needed, or they moved on.
2. **They planned for success.** Their business and marketing plans were living documents and they managed their finances extraordinarily well.
3. **They shared.** They communicated their vision, goals and plans with those important to them, and they researched their clients and stakeholders constantly to learn how to do things better *together*.
4. **They listened.** They listened to their staff, their families and their clients. Then, and only then, when they understood their issues, fears, needs and desires did they offer a solution.
5. **They started smart.** When employing others, whether on contract or as salaried staff, they hired the right people for the right job, and employed people who were strong in areas they were not. When skill gaps appeared, they gave their people the training, systems, environment and recognition to do their job well.

6. **They took calculated risks.** They always looked before they leapt, but they leapt nonetheless. Courage and confidence was something they built as they went.
7. **They believed in themselves, or faked it!** Even professionals doubt themselves– but they don't let self-doubt win.

"You have to believe in yourself. Even when you don't, you have to try," encourages Serena Williams, tennis super-star and 23-time Grand Slam champion.

"There are moments when I am on the court and I'm like, 'I don't think I'm going to be able to do this'. But then I fortify myself and say, 'I can, I can'–and it happens. If you believe in yourself, even if other people don't, that really permeates through and it shows. And people respect that."

If the strategies above sound like things you can do, or are willing to try, chances are self-employment is right for you. But to double check, try the following Entrepreneurial Personality Quiz.

THE ENTREPRENEURIAL
PERSONALITY QUIZ

Do you have the right personality to be an entrepreneur? Are you better suited to becoming a Franchisee? Would contracting suit you better? Or is paid employment really the best option after all?

Before committing yourself to starting your own business of any type, you need to ask yourself whether you have what it takes.

The following quiz is written as though you are still in a salaried role. If you have already started your own business, respond to the questions as though you are still in your last job. Answer as you really are, not how you would like to be.

1. Is accomplishing something meaningful with your life important to you?

2. Do you typically set both short and long-term goals for yourself?
3. Do you usually achieve your goals?
4. Do you enjoy working on your own?
5. Do you like to perform a variety of tasks in your job?
6. Are you self-disciplined?
7. Do you like to be in control of your working environment?
8. Do you take full responsibility for your successes and failures?
9. Are you in excellent physical, mental, and emotional health?
10. Do you have the drive and energy to achieve your goals?
11. Do you have work experience in the type of business you wish to start?
12. Have you ever been so engrossed in your work that time passed unnoticed?
13. Do you consider 'failures' as opportunities to learn and grow?
14. Can you hold to your ideas and goals even when others disagree with you?
15. Are you willing to take moderate risks to achieve your goals?
16. Can you afford to lose the money you invest in your business?

17. When the need arises, are you willing to do a job that may not interest you?
18. Are you willing to work hard to acquire new skills?
19. Do you usually stick with a project until it is completed?
20. Does your family support and stand by you in everything you do?
21. Are you organized and methodical in your work?
22. Does it frustrate you when you can't buy the things you want?
23. Do you like taking calculated gambles?
24. Would you still want your own business, even if there were plenty of other good jobs?
25. Are you a people person?
26. Do you handle personal finances well?
27. As an employee did you/do you regularly suggest new ideas at various levels?
28. Do you feel that you can truly shape your own destiny?
29. How flexible are you when approaching work tasks? If things become difficult do you adapt and complete the task?
30. Is the money you could make one of the primary reasons for starting your own business?

Scoring:

Your answers to at least 20 of these questions should be yes if you are to be successful as a business owner.

The more 'yes' answers, the more likely you are to enjoy the entrepreneurial life and be successful as a business owner.

It is not necessary to answer yes to each of these questions, but if you answer no to some of them you will want to evaluate what that means to you and how significantly it may impact your ability to run your own business.

SUCCESS STORY: A FORK IN THE ROAD

Sheree Clark followed her enthusiasm—her passion for helping others and sharing what she had learned through her own life challenges led her to start her coaching business.

The seeds of change were also cultivated during a stressful time in her life and her former job. She shares her journey of mid-life career reinvention below:

"My current business is Fork in the Road. I am a healthy living (life) coach. I chose the name initially because I was focused on food and healthful eating, and since "fork" conjures up the idea of eating, it seemed to fit. I also believe that at any given point we are all at a proverbial fork in the road.

That fork can be a major one—such as a career choice or the decision to enter or leave a marriage—or a small one, like whether to say yes to dessert or being on another committee. So, when the focus of my business shifted to life coaching for women over 40, the name was still (and perhaps even more) fitting for my practice.

Fork in the Road is truly a crescendo of all of my life experience. I work with my clients to transform their health, reclaim vitality and mental focus, and help ensure they gain clarity on their vision and purpose. These are all things I have done for myself over the course of the last 6+ decades of life.

Deciding what to do

My first business was a marketing communications (advertising) agency that I was "talked into" co-founding in 1985 by a (then) new boyfriend. The truth is, I had grown bored at my job at a local university and had even announced my resignation, effective the following academic year (long notices are an accepted practice at US academic institutions). In the meantime, I had met—and fallen in love with—my later-to-be business partner, and the rest fell into place.

He convinced me that my skill set as a teacher, advisor and mentor would transfer easily to the business development aspect of running an advertising agency. We stayed business partners for 25 years (although the romantic aspect tanked after the initial 14 years).

My current business began after I decided to leave the agency world and (my now-ex) behind.

During my time owning the agency, I had taken a variety of classes simply out of an interest in personal development. Many of the courses had to do with health, nutrition and emotional maturity.

Eventually, as I became less interested in the marketing work and more involved in the business of human potential, it became harder to rally enthusiasm for owning an agency.

Finally, just as we were preparing to commemorate 25 years in business together, I told my partner I wanted to exit our partnership to begin something new.

At that point, I still wasn't certain what my new work would look like, but I knew it wasn't fair to anyone (most especially me!) to stay where I knew I was no longer fully engaged.

So, in essence, I quit—and then I figured it out.

Finding an idea that would be successful— ask your way to success

I found the right product for the right market by trial and error! Next to creating a vision board, the informational interview is my favorite tool for helping me get back on track when I'm feeling lost.

When I was feeling unfulfilled in my business I scheduled a series of interviews with fellow entrepreneurs. I picked women who owned businesses. The only thing they had in common was that I really respected them, even though some I had never met in person.

One of my interviews was with the publisher of a local business newspaper: a fabulous lady who is probably 20 years my senior. We had our meeting over lunch and I told her, candidly, about my inner feelings. I told her I was hoping she might shed some light.

I asked her what she thought my skill

sets and offerings were and where I might be able to plug the gaps. Her feedback? She said she had always thought of me as a teacher and a coach. She said she saw me as articulate, smart and capable, (which in itself is nice to hear, especially coming from someone you admire).

And then she offered up a casual suggestion. She said, "You've always had a way with words. Why don't you write a column for a publication in your industry or some area of your life that brings you joy." Well, that was an idea that resonated, and if nothing else was worth seeing if I could make happen.

The payoff

I went back to my office and sent a query letter to the editor of a graphic design magazine I had written for once or twice before, and asked if they were looking for writers.

Within an hour my phone rang. It was the editor himself. His words nearly knocked me off my chair. He said, "Wow, what timing! We are starting a business advice column in the next quarter, wanna write it?"

I ended up writing that column for five years. Not only did it help scratch an itch I was feeling, I made some extra money in the process. Now, I am not saying you'll have such epic results. But I do know that I have never had an informational interview without a payoff, even if it was just that I got to know somebody a little better.

Working your offerings into your own area of genius

It's not just about finding the right products and services, it's also about working your offerings into your own area of genius.

At this point in my life, while I enjoy making a good income, it's not only about maximizing revenue. I want to do work that brings me joy. I want to work with clients who are a fit for me, so that when I look at my calendar/schedule, I feel excitement, rather than dread.

In my instance, I am what we call a "Baby Boomer" (defined in the USA as being those born between 1946 and 1965). My generation and those slightly after, are all experiencing some major life challenges right now. Our jobs are changing or we've been laid off or deemed "redundant."

Our marriages and family structures are shifting or crumbling: we may suddenly become caretakers or divorcees or widows. Hell, our own bodies are changing and often it feels as though they are betraying us. And for many women over 40, after putting the needs of others first for much of our lives, we can finally say, "it's MY turn now."

What I just described is my area of genius. It's the arena I do best in and it's where I feel most at home. Having for the most part successfully navigated the challenges of being a 40, 50, 60-year old, I get to share my secrets and techniques with other women.

Starting fresh—financing a new career

In both cases when I started my companies I left what I had been doing to embark on the new thing. In the first instance (co-founding the agency) I felt safe doing so because I had a partner and so my risk/exposure was shared.

In the second instance (becoming a coach), I had the luxury of having built savings from the first endeavor, so I could plunge into the second. I recognize that not everyone will have such good fortune.

In both cases, I didn't need any start-up capital.

If I were to give advice, I'd say that while of course you have to consider your own financial situation, also take stock of your risk tolerance.

Entrepreneurship is not certain. There are all sorts of risks and no guarantees. If a lack of financial uncertainty makes you nervous, it's certainly safer to ease into being a business owner, but it can also be more challenging. There are only so many hours in a day!

Finding the confidence to leave the security of a regular salary

It wasn't confidence that propelled me into my second business. It was the pain of not living authentically.

It would be an understatement to say that to close the ad agency I had co-founded was not a decision my former partner and I made easily or lightly. For almost half our lives we had been partners and close friends. But the time had come and we each wanted to do other things with our lives.

I had found a passion in the health and nutrition arena after receiving my certifications as a raw vegan chef and nutrition counselor.

My business partner discovered a love of fine art, and a desire to work more independently. Quite frankly, we both had become rather miserable in our roles as principals and we each needed new challenges.

Despite my excitement for my new future I struggled to dismantle what we had so carefully created. At the time, we decided to close the agency, it was still healthy but my partner's and my passions were on life support.

There were many signs that it was time for a change. I started to dread the out of town travel for clients that I had once so loved. He began to come into the office later and leave earlier.

We both had less patience for employee mistakes and client indecision. For me the defining moment came on a Sunday at church when I actually cried not because the sermon was so moving, but because I knew that in less than 24 hours I had to "go back to work."

It was clearly time to do something.

There are those who have applauded both of us for having the courage to do something so drastic, and others who deem us insane when we could be 'so close to retirement.' All I know is that, as scary as it was, it has rekindled the adrenalin rushes I have not felt in a very, very long time. It was absolutely the right thing to do.

Finding customers

My clients typically follow me online for a period of time before contracting with me for services. Often they run across me because I am a guest speaker at live events, or a subject matter expert on television, or a guest on an online interview series or summit. Others may have been referred to me by a friend or a colleague.

The marketing activities which have been most important and successful for me are speaking and interviews. I also write guest blogs and articles.

Maintaining balance

Running a business should not be a 24/7 thing! Although there are absolutely "push" times, especially in the beginning, I think down time and rest are essential to business success

Down time, time to refuel, is made possible by setting priorities, delegation and hiring (or subcontracting) efficiently. I personally find balance by planning my days the night before.

Each night before I go to bed, I establish what the most important project or priority is for the next day, and that project is the first thing I address after I do my exercise and meditation.

I also find that sometimes I have to actually schedule in my fun times. With my current work schedule, I coach clients the first three weeks of the month.

The last week of every month I take off from individual coaching, and that is when I attend to personal matters such as doing errands, scheduling salon services and meeting friends for social engagements.

I still do work during that fourth week, but because I don't typically schedule client appointments, I have time for other things.

Keeping energy levels high

It's not hard to have high energy when you have high enthusiasm. I love what I do and it keeps me young, vital, engaged and energized. That said, taking care of yourself mentally emotionally and spiritually is also critical. I get adequate sleep, exercise and nutrition. I spend time in nature and in contemplation or prayer.

I have deep relationships. AND I have a coach. That may sound odd, because I AM a coach, but I believe those of us who are most successful, have gotten where we're at with help in identifying blocks, challenges and opportunities. That is what a coach does!

The secret to success, managing cash flow, and generating regular income

For me personally, I have always benefitted from finding and utilizing a good business coach and what is often called a 'mastermind community.' A mastermind is a group of like-minded people who meet regularly to share strategies and tackle challenges and problems together. They lean on each other, give advice, share connections and do business with each other when appropriate.

It's very much peer-to-peer mentoring, and it works! In terms of managing cash flow: one piece of advice is to not take your foot off the 'new business development' gas pedal when you get busy with other things. What you do today will determine your level of success tomorrow.

The learning curve

The biggest learning curve I had was going from owning a company that sold its services in a business to business arena (the communications agency) to one that provided services via a business to consumer model (my coaching practice).

These two ways of conducting business are drastically different. Again, by seeking guidance from peers and by hiring a coach I was able to manage the amount of growing pain.

The best times in my business have usually been the "firsts." First client, first employee, first million-dollar year. The worst have usually been the result of going against my own intuition. Hiring someone I had a gut feeling about because they looked good on paper. Taking a poorly calculated risk because I was listening to my ego instead of looking at the facts or my intuition.

One of the best business books I have

read is, *Turning Pro* by Steven Pressfield. It applies to everyone, but entrepreneurs especially.

What advice would you give to someone who has never started a business or been self-employed?

Start by taking the time to meet with other entrepreneurs and ask them a few questions about things that may have you concerned or sparked your curiosity.

This book, *Mid-Life Career Rescue: Employ Yourself*, is a great start, because it gives you a general 'peek under the tent' at being a business owner, but I would also speak to others in real time.

I often urge my clients to schedule what I refer as an 'informational interview' when they are considering going down new paths or are feeling stuck in some area of their lives.

What are the steps to self-employment? Is there a "right" order?

I have taken the leap to self-employment twice, and each time was different from the other. I think there are too many factors to make a generalized bit of advice valuable here. One caveat I would say to the analytical readers is "don't overthink it."

With my current business, I began by sending a letter to everyone I knew from my former business, telling them what I was transitioning to, and straight-out asking them if they might be interested in my services, or if they would be willing to make a referral. I had enough takers to be encouraged to keep going!

Making the leap sooner

I would have left my first company to start my second company sooner. I was afraid of letting people down: my former partner, my employees, my clients. By the time I left, my passion was on life support.

If I could offer one piece of advice related to starting your own business and employing yourself it would be to know that being an entrepreneur can be lonely sometimes. Your friends, the ones who are employed by others, will think you have it made now.

They will believe that you have all the time in the world to do what you want, and that you're rolling in the money. They'll think you can go on lavish vacations and that you don't have to answer to anyone. Take heart: The other business owners you meet will know the real story.

The secret to self-employed success

Passion. Without it you may be mildly successful, but you'll never be wildly successful!"

Find out more about Sheree's passion-driven business here—www.fork-road.com. Listen to our interviews   here http://www.cassandragaisford.com/media and http://www.cassandragaisford.com/podcast/

I loved, loved, loved what Sheree shared and devoured every word—best of all there were no calories...so that was marvelous. What resonated with you?

Identify and record any lessons can you learn from Sheree's experience of discovering her calling and setting up her business which you could apply to starting your own business. Summarize some possible action steps.

WHAT YOU'VE LEARNED SO FAR

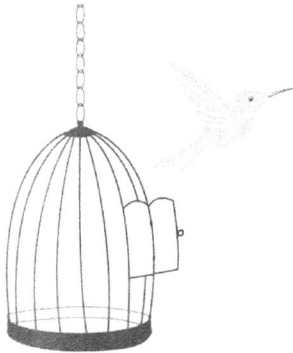

- Before committing yourself to starting your own business or being self-employed, you need to ask yourself whether you have what it takes
- Follow your heart, let your passion and intuition guide you towards the business you were born to create

- You have to believe in yourself—even when you don't
- You don't always need buckets of money, or the courage of a lion, to start your own business. You can start on a shoestring and feel the fear and begin anyway
- Starting a business doesn't have to be a full-time gig. You can start small and keep your current job while you watch your baby grow
- Caring about people and delivering something of value is the key to success

What's Next?

So, now you know the pitfalls of being self-employed and you know some of the joys. But do you really understand what YOU are looking for and why?

The next chapter will help you clarify the motivating forces driving your decisions. Knowing these will help boost your confidence when it comes to making an inspired leap.

WHY DO YOU WANT TO BE YOUR OWN BOSS?

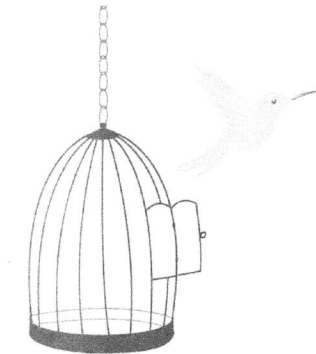

*"Wild horses wouldn't drag me back
to working for someone else."*
Alan Sugar, Entrepreneur and host of The
Apprentice, UK

So now you know the pitfalls of being self-employed and you know some of the joys. But do you really understand what YOU are looking for and why?

Perhaps you can identify with Laura who wants to balance work commitments with caring for her young son. "My boss insists I go to the office. I can't understand why he won't let me work from home."

Do Your Own Thing

Creating your own business is one of the few ways you can generate an income doing what you want, when you want, with whom you want.

It can also be a great way to create an asset—one you can grow and sell later for a profit if you plan things right.

Employing yourself is also a great way to get a job when nobody else will hire you, or when you've lost your job. Like Wendy Pye (her story is shared below), who started her own company and went from redundant to becoming a multi-millionaire.

Running your own business doesn't mean that you are going to be chained to your desk 24/ 7 as some people mistakenly believe. One of the important things prior to starting any new venture is to determine what you want to achieve and why.

. . .

Action Task! Clarify what you really want

Write a list of benefits that self-employment will offer you. If you run out of ideas the following list may help. Identify how you want to feel, and what you want to have, and why this is important to you.

Benefits of Self Employment

Listed below are some of the benefits many people gain from being self-employed. Make a note of those most relevant to you and add these to the list you generated above.

Assess any options you are considering by creating a decision-making criteria checklist. For example, if time freedom is important for you, you may want to reconsider any plans to open a business where people expect you to be there at fixed hours.

- Time freedom—hours to suit yourself
- Flexibility
- No forced retirement age
- Autonomy
- Independence
- Making your own decisions

- Creativity
- Control
- Security—not worrying about corporate layoffs
- Live and work anywhere in the world
- Work from home
- Accountability
- Higher earnings
- Satisfaction and personal fulfillment
- Variety and freedom to be able to work on new ideas and create your own authentic style
- Combine diverse areas of interest, skill and enthusiasm
- Being guided by what feels right in your heart and intuition
- Freedom from financial stress
- Making a difference
- Freedom from the daily grind—a business that runs without you
- Being able to put all your passion and energy into something you believe in, rather than something someone else believes in
- Creating an income producing asset

From Redundant to Multi-Millionaire

Necessity, as some say, is the mother of invention–and often it is the extra push many people need to take a leap into something new.

Some 55,000 New Zealanders are so-called 'necessity entrepreneurs,' people prompted by redundancy or unemployment to set up their own businesses, as distinct from 'opportunity entrepreneurs,' who've become self-employed as a result of planning and choice.

Wendy Pye is the mother of all necessity entrepreneurs. It took a good dose of adversity to get her entrepreneurial juices flowing and she hasn't looked back. She was dumped without warning from NZ News after 22 years with the company, given five minutes to clear her desk, and then marched off the premises.

With no job to go to Pye, then aged 42, set up her own educational publishing company. Now a multi-millionaire, she admits her motivation for going it alone was a desire to show her former employers what she could do.

"I was devastated and disappointed. But it really changed my life, which is a lot better now than if [redundancy] had never happened. I needed the push."

She certainly showed her former employers just what she could do. The 2015 National Business

Review's Rich List, estimates Pye's personal wealth at $105 million.

She has fond thoughts for that executive who laid her off all those years ago. "That guy had vision," she says. "He knew something I didn't know. I can say that and laugh now."

Dubbed one of New Zealand's women power-brokers, Dame Wendy recently won the Business Entrepreneur category in the Women of Influence Awards.

The passion, determination and drive that helped her build her business into one of the most successful education export companies in the world shows no sign of slowing as she heads into her 70s.

Wendy Pye Publishing can now celebrate more than 2000 titles, in more than 20 countries, which have sold over 218 million copies. Her business has also developed digital learning platforms designed to teach children to read and write.

Age is On Your Side

Age is no barrier to employing yourself. Growing numbers of 40-plus men and women are taking up new challenges and starting businesses everyday. Being your own boss gives you more control over your future. If you love what you're doing, chances are you'll never want to retire.

Your life expectancy is on the rise. Which also means you'll be wanting enough money to live comfortably. Employing yourself will help you achieve that.

Ready to learn some new tricks?

As Brian Jones writes in his wonderful book, *Over 50? Start Your Business: Build Wealth, Control Your Destiny. Leave a Legacy*: "Within the last twenty years, technologies such as functional magnetic response imaging (FMRI) have debunked the old-dog-new-tricks myth. Scientists have found that the brain can grow and make new connections at any age. The scientific term for this is neuro-plasticity.

Now more than ever you can be, do and have nearly anything you desire. Like Annie, who aged 54, left teaching and became a romance writer.

Compelling Evidence of Mid-Life Success

Loads of people have employed themselves or started their businesses in mid-life and beyond. Here's just a few:

- Joseph Campbell started Campbell's soup at age 52
- Arianna Huffington started the Huffington post at age 54
- Estee Lauder founded her cosmetics empire when she was 54
- Charles Flint started IBM at 61
- Amadeo Giannini founded the Bank of America when he was 60
- Col. Harlan Sanders launched KFC at age 65
- Heather Morris was 64 when she became a full-time author following her debut success with the publication of *The Tattooist of Auschwitz*

Will you be next? What are you waiting for? If they can do it there's a strong likelihood you can too.

Action Task! Look For Your Heroes

Gather examples of mid-life entrepreneurs who inspire you. Allow them to be your virtual mentors. How can you use their success to guide and encourage you?

WHAT YOU'VE LEARNED SO FAR

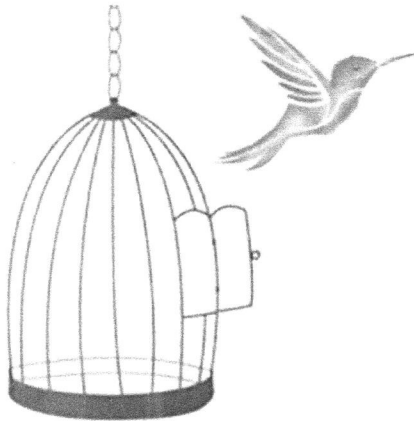

- Intensify your desire, but keep it real. Get clear about what you want to gain by being your own boss and why
- Assess any options you are considering by creating a decision-making criteria checklist

- Sometimes life 'shouts' and gives you the push you need to start your business
- Courageous action can be inspired even at what seems the worst of times. If life is dealing you a raw hand look for opportunities that may be disguised as setbacks
- Age is no barrier to self-employment

What's Next?

Now you have a clearer idea about both your 'what' and your 'why' is, and you have awakened your desire. The next step is to work out exactly what sort of business or self-employment opportunity is right for you.

To do this there is no better place to start than to determine what sets your heart on fire.

PURSUE YOUR PASSION NOT YOUR PENSION

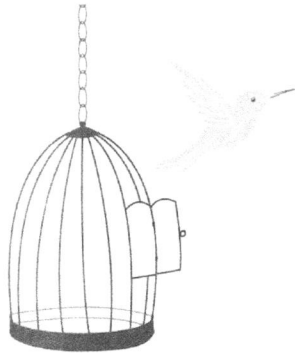

"The starting point of all achievement is desire."
Napoleon Hill, Author

First things first! Start from the heart.
The first and most important commandment of

choosing and growing your business is to follow your passion.

Creating a successful business that you'll love is impossible without passion, enthusiasm, zest, inspiration and the deep satisfaction that comes from doing something that delivers you some kind of buzz.

Passion is a source of energy from the soul, and when you combine it with a product or service that benefits others, that's where you'll find your magic.

Kevin Roberts, former CEO of global advertising agency Saatchi and Saatchi, passionately believes that love is the way forward for business.

Meeting peoples' needs, hopes, dreams, and desires, or offering something which helps them solve problems for which they'd love a cure, is good for people and it's good for business.

"For great brands to survive, they must create Loyalty Beyond Reason," he writes in his book *Lovemarks: The Future Beyond Brands*. Roberts argues, with a ton of facts, and emotionally evocative images to support his premise, that traditional branding practices have become stultified. What's needed are customer Love affairs. "The secret," he maintains, "is the use of Mystery, Sensuality, and Intimacy."

Other experts such as Simon Sinek, author of the bestselling book *Start With Why*, and Robert

Kiyosaki entrepreneur and author of the *Rich Dad, Poor Dad* books, may urge you to begin with rational, head-based logic.

I'm advocating a similar, albeit less analytical approach to begin with. But the premise is similar, to create something meaningful for yourself, and for the customers and clients you wish to attract, you must believe in what you are doing. Your business idea must matter. You must know *why* it's important—to yourself and to others.

"'*Why*' is not money or profit—these are always the results. Why does your organization exist? Why does it do the things it does? Why do customers really buy from one company or another?" challenges Sinek in his book.

I would add, *what* is its purpose? Roberts, would add, *how* can you make them fall in love with you and inspire loyalty beyond reason?

How to Find Your *Why*

When you discover and tap into your passion, you'll find your *why*. You'll also find a huge source of untapped potential that seems to be fearless and knows no bounds. Pursuing your passion in business is profitable on many levels.

Firstly, when you do what you love, this is most

likely where your true talent lies, so you'll stand out in your field. Passion cannot be faked.

Secondly, you will be more enthusiastic about your pursuits. You will have more energy and tenacity to overcome obstacles, and more drive and determination to make things happen.

When you do what you care most about and believe in with such a passion, your work will be not something that you endure, but something that you enjoy. More importantly, work will become a vehicle for self-expression.

Thirdly, passion attracts. As multi-millionaire businesswoman Anita Roddick once said, *'We communicate with passion and passion sells.'*

Ms Roddick founded her company, The Body Shop, on one simple premise—beauty products tested on animals was cruel, barbaric, unnecessary and immoral. Millions of men and women around the world agreed.

People like to do business with people who are passionate about their products and services. When global financial services company KPMG re-branded with passion as a core theme, profitability soared. Check out my presentation on Slideshare to find out how:

http://www.slideshare.net/CassandraGaisford/passionslides-with-kpmg-slides

. . .

Hearts on Fire

The key to sound business planning begins from the inside out. First you need to determine who you are, who you want to be, and what you want to contribute to the world. In working this out, there is no better place to start than with finding out what sets you heart on fire and *why*.

Michael Jr. Comedy, a stand-up comedian and author, explains how discovering your *why* helps you develop options that enable you to live and work with purpose.

"When you know your *why*, you have options on what your *what* can be. For instance, my *why* is to inspire people to walk in purpose. My *what* is stand-up comedy. My *what* is writing books.... Another *what* that has moved me toward my *why* is a web series that we have out now called Break Time."

Check out this clip from one of Michael's most successful episodes http://bit.ly/1PnOTrH. You'll see how working with passion and purpose awakens dormant talents and enables souls to fly higher.

"When you know your *why* your *what* has more impact because you are walking toward your purpose," says Michael.

. . .

We'll dive deeper into discovering your life purpose in the following chapter.

Surf the Web

http://www.eofire.com: Fuel your inspiration by checking out this top-ranked business Podcast where some of the most inspiring entrepreneurs are interviewed 7-days a week. Founder and host John Lee Dumas shares his journey from frustrated employee to inspired entrepreneur via video here http://www.eofire.com/about/

Discovering Your Passion

Everyone is capable of passion; some people just need help taking it out of the drawer. Look for the clues. Often this involves noticing the times you feel most energized and alive, or when you experience a surge of adrenaline through your body.

Sometimes it's the moments when time seems to fly. Perhaps it is something you love to do and would willingly do for free.

Passion is not always about love. The things that push your buttons can lead you to the things that you're most passionate about.

Working long hours, too much stress, financial

strain or a whole raft of other constant pressures can soon send you drowning in a sea of negativity —killing your passion and robbing you of the energy and positivity you need to make a life-enhancing change.

IIf stress is taking a toll on your life you may want to check out the first book in the *Mid-Life Career Rescue* series, *The Call For Change*.

The strategies and tips in the book will help you restore the balance and get your mojo back. You'll also learn how to boost your ability to generate ideas to get unstuck. Available on Amazon in paperback and eBook by clicking the following link >> getBook.at/CareerChange

If you need more help to you manage stress my book, *Stress Less. Love Life More: How to Stop Worrying, Reduce Anxiety, Eliminate Negative Thinking and Find Happiness*, available as a paperback and eBook will help. Navigate to here—getBook.at/StressLess.

Action Task! Find Your Passion

Real passion is more than a fad or a fleeting enthusiasm. It can't be turned on and off like a light switch. Answering the following questions will help you begin to clarify the things you are most passionate about:

1. **When does time seem to fly?** When was the last time you felt really excited, or deeply absorbed in, or obsessed by something? What were you doing? Who were you with? What clues did you notice?
2. **What do you care deeply or strongly about?** Discovering all the things that you believe in is not always easy. Look for the clues to your deep beliefs by catching the times you use words such as 'should' or 'must.'
3. **What do you value?** What do you need to experience, feel, or be doing to feel deeply fulfilled?
4. **What pushes your buttons or makes you angry?** How could you use your anger constructively to bring about change?
5. **Which skills and talents come most easily or naturally to you?** Which skills do you love using? What skills do you look forward to using? What gives you such a buzz or a huge sense of personal satisfaction that you'd keep doing it even if you weren't paid?
6. **What inspires you?** To be inspired is to be in spirit. What bewitches and

enthralls you so much that you lose all track of time? What makes your soul sing? What floats your boat? What things, situations, people, events etc. fill you with feelings of inspiration? List all your obsessions and the things that interest you deeply. If you're struggling to identify your interests and inspirations, you'll find some handy prompts in the next chapter.

7. **Keep a passion journal.** My passion is passion—to help others live and work with passion and to bring about positive change in the world. If you're not sure what you are passionate about, creating a passion journal is one simple but powerful technique to help achieve clarity. Your passion journal is where manifesting your preferred future really happens. I've been keeping a passion journal for years and so many things I've visualized and affirmed on the pages, are now my living realities—personally and professionally.

Love Is Where The Magic Is

Love is where the magic is. When you love what you do with such a passion you'd do it for free this is your path with heart. You've heard the saying, 'when you do what you love, you'll never work again.' It's true. Work doesn't feel like a slog, it feels energizing.

As Annie Featherston, writing as Sophia James, shared in the second book on the *Mid-Life Career Rescue* series, *What Makes You Happy*, "When you combine your favorite skills with doing something you completely and utterly love, you come home to your True Self and find your place of bliss. The result? Contentment—and more often than not, producing something highly marketable."

Passion in Business

A good way to find your own passion and identify ways to turn it into a fulfilling self-employment opportunity is to look for examples of others who have started businesses they are passionate about.

Here are just a few of many examples:

A passion for bugs! Brian Clifford is passionate about helping people and bugs. He has combined his passion into a successful business as a pest controller.

"All the rats, all the maggots, all the cockroaches all over the place, these are the things that I love doing,' he says. His business motto is, 'If it bugs you, I'll kill it!"

Check out his business here >> www.borercontrolwellington.co.nz

A passion for bones! John Holley has turned his passion for bones into a business, Skulls Down Under, selling skeletons to museums all over the world.

Check out his business here >> www.skullsdownunder.co.nz

A passion for Maori food. Charles Royal's passion for finding a way to incorporate traditional Maori foods into modern dishes led him to start his own business—Kinaki Wild Herbs.

"I had learned a lot about the bush during my time in the army and have taken that knowledge through the years, developing food tours and cooking classes using what we gather from the wild. I love organics and making something out of nothing, but you have to know what you are looking for," says Royal. Air New Zealand now serves pikopiko and horopito in its First and Business Classes.

Check out his business here >> www.maori-food.com

SUCCESS STORY: A LOVE OF GOOD FOOD

"Passion is Everything—If You Don't Have It You Will Not Succeed"

A love of good food and a lifelong dream to open their passion-driven business in London fueled Wellington restauranteurs Vivienne Haymans and Ashley Sumners' move to the UK.

"We both felt we had gone as far as we could with our business in New Zealand and wanted to move further afield," says Vivienne.

"I came here for a three-month holiday, secretly wanting to stay longer and build a business overseas. On arriving I discovered that London seriously needed a restaurant like our Sugar Club in Wellington. There was nowhere in

London doing anything like it. I called Ash and a year later he also moved to London after selling our Wellington restaurant."

They relocated the restaurant to Notting Hill in 1995, then to Soho in 1998, winning the Time Out "Best Modern British Restaurant" award in 1996 and "Best Central London Restaurant" award in 1999, along with several Evening Standard Eros awards.

Since then they have expanded and diversified their restaurant business, opening a chain of modern *traiteurs* (Italian-style delicatessens) that offer delicious, easy-to-prepare hand-made meals and great New Zealand coffee.

The first of these is called The Grocer on Elgin, situated in the heart of Notting Hill. Vivienne designed all three restaurants and 'The Grocer On' stores.

Like many people following their passion, Vivienne and Ash faced significant barriers before finally making it big.

"It took Ash and I seven years to fulfill our dream of opening The Sugar Club in London. When we first arrived there were huge premiums being asked for restaurant sites.

Then, with the early 90s recession they were giving restaurants away but, like now, the banks were not lending. We had no property assets at the time, limited funds, a reference from our NZ lawyer, accountant and bank manager and a handful of NZ press clippings. The banks wanted property assets and UK business records. No less."

Just when it looked like the obstacles were insurmountable, their passion for great food and design, the quality of the produce, and the integrity of its production, produced lucky fruit.

"We were offered a site by a landlord that we had had dealings with in the past. He liked what we did and gave us the lease. We developed the old Singapore Pandang into the Notting Hill Sugar Club. I borrowed an extra £5000 from my mum and paid her back in a month. It was an instant success and well worth the long wait."

Vivienne says that following their passion is an important ingredient in their success.

"Passion is everything—if you don't have it you will not succeed. It is hard work; your passion will pull you through the seriously bad times, which will always occur."

Hot Tip! Gathering your own examples of passionate people and businesses is a great way to build confidence and generate your own business ideas.

Here are some things that other people who are self-employed are passionate about:

- **Creating Businesses**—Entrepreneurs Melissa Clarke Reynolds and Eric Watson
- **Airports**—Graham is an airport designer
- **Boats**—Bill Day runs a specialist maritime service business
- **Beauty**—Joy Gaisford, Designer
- **Food**—Ruth Pretty, Caterer and food writer
- **Astronomy**—Richard Hall, Stonehenge Aotearoa
- **Design**—Luke Pierson, runs a web design business
- **Rocks**—Carl created Carlucciland—a rock-themed amusement park
- **Passion**—Cassandra Gaisford helping people work and live their passion!

Here are some things that some businesses are passionate about:

- **Animal Welfare and Human Rights**—The Body Shop
- **Technology**—Microsoft, Apple
- **Helping people**—Worklife Solutions, Venus Network
- **Equality**—The EEO Trust, and the Johnstone Group
- **The Environment**—The Conservation Department
- **Honey**—The Honey Hive
- **Chocolate**—Chocaholic
- **Pampering Others**—East Day Spa

Tune In To Your Body Barometer

What pushes your buttons or makes you angry? Having my manager threaten to 'smash my head in,' and working with others who were bullies and tyrants, the relentless pursuit of profit at the expense of caring for people, and numerous work restructurings, motivated me to gain my independence.

That and getting shingles—something I wrote

about in my first books, *The Call for Change*, and also *What Makes You Happy.*

Shingles was definitely my body barometer sending me a red alert! As was seeing my colleagues suffer heart attacks.

As Neale Walsch, the author of *Conversations with God*, says, "Judge not about which you feel passionate. Simply notice it, then see if it serves you, given who and what you wish to be."

So, as I've mentioned earlier, rather than become bitter, I thought how could I use my anger constructively to bring about change?

I decided I wanted to help people find jobs that made them happy, and I wanted to help victims of workplace bullying. That was my *why* and my *what*.

Stepping Stones to Success

I started a career counseling business for an established workplace counseling organization before going out on my own.

Working as an employee first gave me the confidence to fly free. I became more motivated when the CEO changed and the new boss tried to manage me. Increasingly, the job began to frustrate me.

It lacked challenge, my salary was capped, and I was finding it increasingly difficult to balance childcare. The final clincher however was when I did the math.

I worked out my hourly rate as a full-time salaried employee, versus what they charged me out per hour, and how much business I was bringing in for them, and came to the conclusion they were buying my skills, but they weren't paying me enough. I could work less and earn and achieve more if I employed myself. I started to feel excited!

Action Task! Tune into Your Body Barometer

Notice the times you feel strong emotions. These could be annoyance, irritation and anger. Or they could be a sense of excitement, a state of arousal, a feeling of limitless energy, a burning desire, a strong gut feeling, a feeling of contentment or determination. Notice these feelings and record them in your passion journal.

Go deeper. Ask, "How could I make a living from my passion?" or "How do others make a living from things that excite or motivate me?"

Explore possibilities. Even a simple Google search, or generating ideas with others could get you started down the right path.

** FREE BONUS **

If you haven't downloaded the free copy of the Passion Workbook, download it here >>http://worklifesolutions.leadpages.co/free-find-your-passion-workbook.

WHAT YOU'VE LEARNED SO FAR

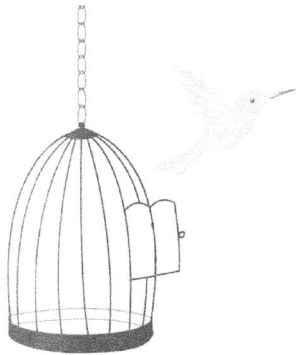

- Passion is energy. It is emotion, zest, intensity, enthusiasm and excitement. Passion is love
- Creating more love in the world is the way forward for business. Meeting peoples' needs, hopes, dreams and desires, or offering something which

helps them solve problems for which they'd love a cure, is good for people and its good for business

- Do what moves you. Pursuing your passion, not your pension, can be a liberating and clarifying catalyst to your true calling and the business you were born to create

- A healthy obsession can lead to many things. Not only will your passion lead you to your path with heart, it will also help fuel the fires of determination, courage and self-belief. You'll be fully alive, stand out from the crowd and gain a competitive edge

- If you don't know where to look, passion can be difficult to find. Tune into your body barometer and notice the times when you feel most alive, inspired or fulfilled

- Start a passion journal—keep track of the times when you notice clues to your passion, such as a feeling of inspiration or any of the other signs discussed in this chapter. Record these moments so that they don't get lost or forgotten

- Adding quotes, pictures or any other insights will really make your journal come alive. Gain greater awareness of what drives your passion by asking yourself, "Why am I passionate about this?" Look for the themes and patterns that build up over time

- Keep your passion alive by updating your journal and referring to it regularly. Actively look for examples of people who have made the things you are passionate about into a rewarding business

What's Next?

In the next chapter you'll discover how joyous and exciting work and life is when you're working with a higher purpose.

Did you enjoy this excerpt?
    Grab The Ultimate Guide to Freedom
    Mid-Life Career Rescue: Employ Yourself
    Start a business on the side while holding down your job. Or take the leap to self-employed bliss. Choose and grow your own business with confidence. This handy resource will show you how.
    Available in print and eBook.

DID YOU ENJOY THIS EXCERPT?

If you need more help and a step-by-step guide to becoming your own boss my book, *Employ Yourself*, available as a paperback and eBook from Amazon will help. Navigate to here getBook.at/EmployYourself

To fuel the flames of inspiration to help you create a passion and purpose inspired business, The Passion-Driven Business Planning Journal:The Effortless Path to Manifesting Your Business and Career Goals, available as a paperback and eBbook from Amazon will help. Navigate to here viewBook.at/PassionBusinessJournal

Or you may prefer to take my online course, and watch inspirational and practical videos and other strategies to help you to fulfil your potential —https://the-coaching-lab.teachable.com/p/ follow-your-passion-and-purpose-to-prosperity.

AFTERWORD

I hope you have found a few useful tips in this book to help you control anxiety, conquer stress and fuel greater resilience. Mastering the ability to slay toxic stress dragons lies at the heart of your mental, emotional, spiritual, and physical well-being.

I always believe that I should practice what I preach and so you can be sure that many of the strategies and techniques I have shared with you are ones I have put into practice myself. Writing this book is a case in point. It really was a case of putting all that I knew into practice—once again.

This book is a labor of love, passion, and purpose. One that had its seeds in the culmination and intersection of my talents, my interests, my motivations, and external drivers. Life kept telling me that this was a book I not only wanted to write but was called to write.

Requests from my readers and also from clients provided a compelling reminder to crack on and finish this book.

External factors also spurred my motivation, like juggling work, running multiple businesses, supporting my partner through family dramas—and then, as if I wasn't "stressed" enough, a toxic, narcissistic employer stole what little peace of mind I had managed to salvage.

So, yes—life is stressful. Sometimes exceedingly stressful. There's so much and so many people lining up to feed your anxiety—if you let them. I've discovered first-hand just how essential it is to build resilience ahead of time. I hope you have, too.

I've also learned to revalue the spiritually-motivating power of living to a purpose and strengthened my intuitive powers in the process.

I've been inspired by the American singer, Meatloaf. His mission to find a producer for his album *Bat Out of Hell* is such an inspirational story about passion, grit, perseverance, failure, and ultimate success.

Plus, I've followed one of my muses, Richard Branson, whose wise words, "If it's not fun I'm not doing it," have reminded me to always work with joy.

Follow Your Joy

What is my joy? Well, I have several, but one of the most important is that by writing this book I have helped you gain the clarity, confidence, courage and inspiration to live a happy, healthy life and to follow your dreams.

I dream that you, and those you love, can be truly happy, and that your happiness will spread the seeds of joy amongst all you meet.

I dream that one day the current research that states that less than 80% of people are suffering from anxiety will be surpassed by new data showing that over 80% of people are happy at work and in life.

Is this really dreaming? Decide for yourself. Perhaps, this book will help you to turn your dreams of a happy working life into a fulfilling reality.

Thank you for allowing me to go on this journey with you. Stay optimistic—you can handle anything that comes your way.

Passionately and happily yours,
Cassandra

P.S. What feeds your spirit?

I feel passionately about spiritually approaches

to healing. As one of my clients, a 10-year-old boy who I taught to meditate as part of his anxiety, and anger cure, said to me,

"Thanks for meditating with me. It was like being on another planet."

In response to this feedback, I wrote a second book in *The Anxiety Cure* series called, *Love Your Soul.*

In *Love Your Soul,* I'll help you clarify what you need to feel happy, enriched with purpose, and to be fulfilled. Plus we'll dive deeper into discovering your vein of gold—the strengths, gifts and natural talents you have to give the world.

If you'd like to be the first to know when this and other books become available, sign up for my newsletter and receive free giveaways, sneak peeks into new books and helpful tips and strategies to live life more passionately.

Mid-Life Career Rescue:

The Call for Change
What Makes You Happy
Employ Yourself
Job Search Strategies That Work
3 Book Box Set: The Call for Change, What Makes You Happy, Employ Yourself
4 Book Box Set: The Call for Change, What Makes You Happy, Employ Yourself, Job Search Strategies That Work

The Art of Living:

How to Find Your Passion and Purpose

How to Find Your Passion and Purpose Companion Workbook
Career Rescue: The Art and Science of Reinventing Your Career and Life
Boost Your Self-Esteem and Confidence

Journaling Prompts Series:

The Passion Journal
The Passion-Driven Business Planning Journal
How to Find Your Passion and Purpose 2 Book-Bundle Box Set

Health & Happiness:

Anxiety Rescue
The Happy, Healthy Artist
Stress Less. Love Life More
Bounce: Overcoming Adversity, Building Resilience and Finding Joy
Bounce Companion Workbook

Mindful Sobriety:

Mind Your Drink: The Surprising Joy of Sobriety
Mind Over Mojitos: How Moderating Your Drinking Can Change Your Life:Easy Recipes for Happier Hours & a Joy-Filled Life

Your Beautiful Brain: Control Alcohol and Love Life More

Happy Sobriety:
Happy Sobriety: Non-Alcoholic Guilt-Free Drinks You'll Love
The Sobriety Journal
Happy Sobriety Two Book Bundle-Box Set: Alcohol and Guilt-Free Drinks You'll Love & The Sobriety Journal

Money Manifestation:

Financial Rescue: The Total Money Makeover: Create Wealth, Reduce Debt & Gain Freedom

The Prosperous Author:

Developing a Millionaire Mindset
Productivity Hacks: Do Less & Make More
Two Book Bundle-Box Set (Books 1-2)

Miracle Mindset:

Change Your Mindset: Millionaire Mindset Makeover: The Power of Purpose, Passion, & Perseverance

More of Cassandra's practical and inspiring work-books on a range of career and life enhancing topics can be found on her website (www. cassandragaisford.com) and her author page at all good online bookstores.

FOLLOW YOUR PASSION TO PROSPERITY ONLINE COURSE

If you need more help to find and live your life purpose you may prefer to take my online course, and watch inspirational and practical videos and other strategies to help you fulfill your potential.

Follow your passion and purpose to prosperity—online coaching program

Easily discover your passion and purpose, overcoming barriers to success, and create a job or business you love with my self-paced online course.

Gain unlimited lifetime access to this course, for as long as you like—across any and all devices you own. Be supported with practical, inspirational, easy-to-access strategies to achieve your dreams.

To start achieving outstanding personal and professional results with absolute certainty and excitement. **Click here to enroll or find out more— https://the-coaching-lab.teachable.com/p/ follow-your-passion-and-purpose-to-prosperity**

FURTHER RESOURCES

SURF THE NET

www.bornthisway.foundation

Founded by Lady Gaga to empower youth, inspire bravery and encourage kindness. Offers inspiration, support, and research to promote mental health.

Mathew Johnstone has a wide range of books and resources on mental wellness and mindfulness: www.matthewjohnstone.com.au

Brad Yates shares a wonderful way to self-help your way through anxiety to self-love in his YouTube videos. You can check it one of them here —https://youtu.be/K6kq9N9Yp6E

www.whatthebleep.com—a powerful and inspiring site emphasizing quantum physics and the transformational power of thought.

www.heartmath.org—comprehensive information and tools help you access your intuitive insight and heart-based knowledge. Validated and supported by science-based research. Check out the additional information about your heart-brain.

Join polymath Tim Ferris and learn from his interesting and informative guests on The Tim Ferris Show http://fourhourworkweek.com/podcast/.

Listen to podcasts which inspire you to become the best version of your writing self—*Joanna Penn's podcast* is very helpful for "authorpreneurs" http://www.thecreativepenn.com/podcasts. I also love Neil Patel's podcast for savvy marketing strategies http://neilpatel.com/podcast.

Experience the transformative power of hypnosis. One of my favorite hypnosis sites is the UK-based Uncommon Knowledge. On their website http://www.hypnosisdownloads.com you'll find a range of self-hypnosis mp3 audios, including The Millionaire Mindset program.

Celebrity hypnotherapist and author Marissa Peer is another favorite source of subconscious re-programming and liberation—www.marisapeer.com.

What beliefs are holding you back? Check out Peer's Youtube clip "How To Teach Your Mind That Everything Is Available To You" here —https://www.youtube.com/watch?v=IKeaAbM2kJg

Enjoy James Clear's fabulous blog content and receive further self-improvement tips based on proven scientific research: http://jamesclear.com/articles

Tim Ferriss recommends a couple of apps for those wanting some help getting started with meditation —Headspace (www.headspace.com) or Calm (www.calm.com).

National Geographic: The Science of Stress: Portrait of a killer
https://www.youtube.com/watch?v=ZyBsy5SQxqU

Effects of Stress on Your Body
https://www.youtube.com/watch?v=1p6EeYwp1O4

Mindfulness training

Wellington-based Peter Fernando offers an introductory guided meditation which you can take further. He also meets with individuals and groups in Wellington for philosophical talks on mindfulness and Buddhism. Very enjoyable and great for the soul.

http://www.monthofmindfulness.info

Guided meditations

www.calm.com

Free app with guided meditations

http://eocinstitute.org/meditation/emotional-benefits-of-meditation/

Includes a comprehensive list of the benefits of meditation.

Career Guidance Sites:

www.aarp.org/work - information and tools to help you stay current and connected with what's hot and what's not in today's workplace.

www.lifereimagined.org - loads of inspiration and practical tips to help you maximize your interests and expertise, personalized and interactive.

www.personalitytype.com—created by the authors of *Do What You Are: Discover the Perfect Career for You through the Secrets of Personality Type.* This site focuses on expanding your awareness of your own type and that of others—including children and partners. This site also contains many useful links.

BOOKS

Repurpose trauma with Azita Nahai, *Trauma to Dharma: Transform Your Pain into Purpose*

Treatment of Complex Trauma: A Sequenced, Relationship-Based Approach by Christine Courtois and Julian Ford
   Journey Through Trauma: A Trail Guide to the 5-Phase Cycle of Healing Repeated Trauma by Gretchen Schmelzer, PhD

The Complex PTSD Workbook: A Mind-Body Approach to Regaining Emotional Control and Becoming Wholeby Arielle Schwartz, PhD

The Body Keeps Score: Brain, Mind, And Body In The Healing Of Trauma by Bessel van der Kolk

Struggling in an extroverted world? Introverts are enjoying a renaissance, fueled in part by Susan

Cain's terrific bestseller, *Quiet: The Power of Introverts in a World That Can't Stop Talking.*

Roll up your sleeves and bring out the big guns to win your creative battle with *The War of Art* by Steven Pressfield.

Power up with a new personality—read Breaking the Habit of Being Yourself: How to Lose Your Mind and Create a New One by Dr. Joe Dispenza.

Unleash the power of your mind by reading *You Are the Placebo: Making Your Mind Matter,* by Dr. Joe Dispenza.

Manifest your prosperity with Rhonda Byrne in her popular book, *The Secret.*

Ensure you don't starve by reading Jeff Goins collated wisdom in *Real Artists Don't Starve: Timeless Strategies for Thriving in the New Creative Age.*

Fortify your faith with Julia Cameron's book, *Faith and Will.*

How to Survive and Thrive in Any Life Crisis, Dr. Al Siebert

Thrive: The Third Metric to Redefining Success and Creating a Happier Life, Arianna Huffington

(This book has great content throughout and some excellent resources listed in the back.)

The Power of Now: A Guide to Spiritual Enlightenment, Eckhart Tolle

The Book of Joy, The Dalai Lama and Archbishop Desmond Tutu

The Sleep Revolution: Transforming Your Life One Night at a Time, Arianna Huffington

Quiet the Mind: An Illustrated Guide on How to Meditate, Mathew Johnstone

Comfortable with Uncertainty: 108 Teachings on Cultivating Fearlessness and Compassion, Pema Chodron

Power vs. Force: The Hidden Determinants of Human Behavior, David R. Hawkins

Learn how to live an inspired life with Tarot cards and other oracles. Read Jessa Crispin's book, *The Creative Tarot: A Modern Guide to an Inspired Life.*

Check out all of Collette-Baron-Reid's books, including: *Uncharted: The Journey Through Uncertainty to Infinite Possibility* and *Messages from Spirit: The Extraordinary Power of Oracles, Omens, and Signs.*

PLEASE LEAVE A REVIEW

Word of mouth is the most powerful marketing force in the universe. If you found this book useful, I'd appreciate you rating this book and leaving a review. You don't have to say much—just a few words about how the book helped you learn something new or made you feel.

"Your books are a fantastic resource and until now I never even thought to write a review. Going forward I will be reviewing more books. So many great ones out there and I want to support the amazing people that write them."
Great reviews help people find good books.

Thank you so much! I appreciate you!

ABOUT THE AUTHOR

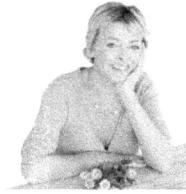

Cassandra Gaisford, is a holistic therapist, award-winning artist, and #1 bestselling author. A corporate escapee, she now lives and works from her idyllic lifestyle property overlooking the Bay of Islands in New Zealand.

Cassandra is best known for the passionate call to redefine what it means to be successful in today's world.

She is a well-known expert in the area of success, passion, purpose and transformational business, career and life change, and is regularly sought after as a keynote speaker, and by media seeking an expert opinion on career and personal development issues.

Cassandra has also contributed to international publications and been interviewed on national radio and television in New Zealand and America.

She has a proven-track record of successfully helping people find savvy ways to boost their finances, change careers, build a business or become a solopreneur—on a shoestring.

Cassandra's unique blend of business experience and qualifications (BCA, Dip Pych.), creative skills, and well-ness and holistic training (Dip Counselling, Reiki Master Teacher) blends pragmatism and commercial savvy with rare and unique insight and out-of-the-box-thinking for anyone wanting to achieve an extraordinary life.

Learn more about her on her website, her blog, or connect with her on Facebook and Twitter.

STAY IN TOUCH

FOLLOW ME AND CONTINUE TO BE INSPIRED

Follow Me And Continue To Be Supported, Encouraged, and Inspired

www.cassandragaisford.com
www.twitter.com/cassandraNZ
www.instagram.com/cassandragaisford
www.youtube.com/cassandragaisfordnz
www.pinterest.com/cassandraNZ
www.linkedin.com/in/cassandragaisford
www.facebook.com/cassandra.gaisford

I invite you to share your stories and experiences in our Career Rescue Community. We'd love to hear from you! To join, visit https://www.facebook.com/Career_Rescue

BLOG

Be inspired by regular posts to help you increase your wellness, follow your bliss, slay self-doubt, and sustain healthy habits.

Learn more about how to achieve happiness and success at work and life by visiting my blog:

www.cassandragaisford.com/archives

SPEAKING EVENTS

Cassandra is available internationally for speaking events aimed at wellness strategies, motivation, inspiration and as a keynote speaker.

She has an enthusiastic, humorous and passionate style of delivery and is celebrated for her ability to motivate, inspire and enlighten.

For information navigate to www.cassandragaisford.com/contact/speaking

To ask Cassandra to come and speak at your workplace or conference, contact: cassandra@cassandragaisford.com

NEWSLETTERS

For inspiring tools and helpful tips subscribe to Cassandra's free newsletters here: http://www.cassandragaisford.com

Sign up now and receive a free eBook to help you find your passion and purpose!

ACKNOWLEDGMENTS

To all the amazingly interesting clients who have allowed me to help them over the years, and to the wonderful people who read my books and wrote to me with their stories of reinvention—thank you. Your feedback, deep sharing, requests for help, and inspired, courageous action continues to inspire me.

A huge thank you also to my amazing proofreader Cate Walker, once again, for your beautiful and thorough editing. I am truly blessed to have received your input and cheerleading.

My thanks also to my terrific friends and supporters. And, of course, I can never say thank you enough to my family, particularly my parents and grandparents, who have instilled me with such tremendous values and life skills.

My daughter, Hannah—I wish for you everything that your heart desires. Without you, I doubt I would ever have accomplished all the things I have in my life.

Thank you.